MASTERING THE ZONE

THE NEXT STEP IN ACHIEVING SUPERHEALTH AND PERMANENT FAT LOSS

Barry Sears, Ph.D.

ReganBooks

An Imprint of HarperCollinsPublishers

HarperCollins books may be purchased for educational, business, or sales promotional use. For information please write: Special Markets Department, HarperCollins Publishers, Inc., 10 East 53rd Street, New York, NY 10022.

FIRST EDITION

Designed by Nancy Singer

Library of Congress Cataloging-in-Publication Data

Sears, Barry, 1947–
    Mastering the zone : the next step in achieving superhealth and permanent fat loss / Barry Sears.
        p.   cm.
    Includes bibliographical references and index.
    ISBN 0-06-039190-1
    1. Weight loss. 2. Nutrition. 3. Health. I. Title.
RM222.2.S389 1997
613.2'5--dc21   96-39111

01 00 99 98 RRD-H 30 29 28 27 26 25 24

CONTENTS

ACKNOWLEDGMENTS

No book is ever written alone, and this book is no exception. First and foremost I want to thank the thousands of individuals who have been using the principles of the Zone over the last several years. Their feedback has been essential in refining the program by identifying pitfalls and offering shortcuts to help make getting into the Zone easier than ever before. Just as important is the patience and support of my family, especially my wife, Lynn Sears, who was instrumental in editing much of this book. Likewise my brother, Doug, who has been my partner and close collaborator over the past fourteen years, as the dietary technology that is the core of the Zone has emerged. Without his support, the concept of the Zone might never have seen the light of day. Special thanks also goes to my first employee, my mother, who finally retired after twenty years of service. She and my brother helped make many of my early concepts take shape into reality. I would also like to thank Sherry Sontag and Jill Sullivan for their valuable editorial comments.

The Zone recipes are the work of Scott C. Lane, who is the Executive Chef and Quality Assurance Manager of one of the major food manufacturing companies in the United States. As a graduate of the Culinary Institute of America and a college instructor in the culinary arts, Scott brings a unique perspective in making great-tasting meals with advanced food technology.

I would be remiss in not thanking Michael and Mary Dan Eades for their fruitful and insightful discussions over the past years about the concept of hyperinsulinemia, and how this medical problem can be addressed at the clinical level. These discussions have significantly helped to refine my dietary concepts on eicosanoid control. More important, we have become extremely close friends during our years together.

My thanks go out as well to Todd Silverstein for his invaluable editorial advice and support and to the rest of the ReganBooks/HarperCollins team for their hard work on this project.

Finally, I wish to thank Judith Regan, my publisher, for her belief in the Zone, and her continued support in bringing the concept to the public.

PREFACE

I hoped that by writing *The Zone,* I would be taking the first step in unearthing the Rosetta Stone of nutrition on how food affects hormonal response. Furthermore, I hoped to provide a readable summary of my work to other medical researchers, as well as to the lay public, who knew very little about those seemingly mystical and almost magical hormones known as eicosanoids that ultimately control our lives. Frankly, I never expected *The Zone* would sell so well. I am gratified, but still overwhelmed by the response. Yet I realize that many readers of *The Zone* still find it difficult to apply the concepts of the Zone to their daily lives. I hope that *Mastering the Zone* will remove many of those barriers, because in reality, the Zone Diet is incredibly easy to follow on a lifetime basis. *Mastering the Zone* is a compilation of the advice I have given over the years on how to easily integrate the principles of the Zone into your own life, whether you're a cardiovascular patient or a world-class athlete, or somewhere between these extremes.

Obviously, I had a strong personal reason for this quest to understand the Zone: my own health. With a family history of early death from heart disease, I knew I couldn't change my genes, but I could possibly control their expression by manipulation of levels of eicosanoids in my body. Frankly, I was willing to bet my life on the Zone.

Now that I'm forty-nine, the obvious question is, how am I doing? Every cardiovascular indicator says that I have the heart of a twenty-five-year-old. More important, I feel I have uncovered a fundamental pathway to achieving SuperHealth that is easy for everyone to follow. What is SuperHealth? In essence, it is doing everything in your power to squeeze as much quality out of life as possible, and in the process begin to dissociate biological age from chronological age.

Writing both books has been like keeping a personal diary of my own scientific journey toward understanding how food controls hormonal response. I never anticipated the twists and turns of that journey, nor the fact it would take me nearly fourteen years to decipher this Rosetta Stone of nutrition. The Zone is not intuitively obvious, but it is based on a combination of cutting-edge biotechnology and common sense.

I hope that after you read this book, you can say the magic phrase, "I can do this," because if you can, you have taken a major step forward to enhance the quality of your life by achieving SuperHealth. And in my opinion, the only way to achieve SuperHealth is by reaching the Zone and staying there on a lifelong basis.

This book is not intended to replace medical advice or be a substitute for a physician. If you are sick or suspect you are sick, you should see a physician. If you are taking a prescription medication, you should never change diet (for better or worse) without consulting your physician, because any dietary change will affect the metabolism of that prescription drug.

Prevention will always be the best medicine. However, prevention can only be undertaken by the individual, and that includes eating correctly. This is the foundation of a healthy lifestyle. You have to eat, so you might as well eat wisely.

Although this book is about food, the author and publisher expressly disclaim responsibility for any adverse effects arising from the use of nutritional supplements to your diet without appropriate medical supervision.

1

YOUR GRANDMOTHER COULD DO IT. WHY CAN'T YOU?

Mastering the Zone. Sounds very New Age, like Yoda teaching Luke Skywalker about the Force. But it's not. Instead it's very similar to the advice your grandmother gave you about eating. Eat everything in moderation, eat lots of fruits and vegetables, and have some protein at every meal. Your grandmother didn't know it, but she was teaching you the basic principles for developing a life-long strategy of hormonal balance. If you can achieve this hormonal balance, you are well on your way to the Zone.

What is the Zone? It is the balance of hormonal responses that occurs every time you eat. A perfect equilibrium: not too high, not too low. Why should you want to get there? Simply said, if you can keep yourself in the Zone, then you will:

A. think better, because in the Zone you are maintaining stable blood sugar levels,
B. perform better, because being in the Zone allows you to increase oxygen transfer to your muscle cells,
C. look better, because in the Zone you are shedding excess body fat at the fastest possible rate, and
D. never be hungry between meals, because staying in the Zone means your brain is being constantly supplied with its primary fuel: blood sugar.

All these benefits of being in the Zone will emerge within a one- to two-week period if you follow the instructions in this book.

But the best reason to want to stay in the Zone on a lifelong basis is to achieve SuperHealth.

For most people, health is defined as the absence of disease. SuperHealth goes beyond that. In a state of SuperHealth you will reduce the likelihood of developing chronic disease, the types of illnesses that represent the bulk of our health care costs. If you have read *The Zone,* you know that SuperHealth is exactly what you are aiming for. And the only way to obtain SuperHealth is to take control of your diet, and use it to keep yourself in the Zone on a continual basis. The more time you spend in the Zone, the more control you have over the ultimate quality of your life.

When I wrote *The Zone* in 1995, I tried to show that the age-old inherent common sense about dietary balance is really cutting-edge twenty-first-century hormonal control technology that can be mathematically defined with a precision your grandmother never dreamed of. While your grandmother's diet was prepared intuitively, you can do it scientifically.

This book marks the next step on that quest. It will show you how to make a wide range of food choices, from gourmet meals to fast-food drive-through fare and everything in between, while still staying in the Zone. Although thinking of food hormonally may be revolutionary, eating in the Zone is not. In fact, eating in the Zone is a lot like eating your grandmother's cooking (except for the fast food).

For those of you already in the Zone, this book offers new information on making the Zone part of your lifelong routine, from tips on eating out and shopping, to information about adjusting the Zone Diet to your own body chemistry, to more than a hundred and fifty new Zone meals that will make it easier for you to stay there. For those of you still struggling to reach the Zone, this volume will make your journey much faster and easier.

Once you use these tips, getting into the Zone and staying there becomes second nature because you will be eating the foods you already like to eat and adapting the recipes you currently use everyday into great Zone meals.

Let me help you visualize the Zone on a plate: a moderate serving of low-fat protein (such as fish or chicken) with a significant amount of vegetables covered with slivered almonds, and fruit for dessert. Every time you eat, make sure that your carbohydrates come with a protein chaser and a dash of fat. To be a little more precise, for every cup of vegetables, or half a piece of fruit or ¼ cup of pasta that you plan to eat (these serving sizes will be explained later on), add an ounce of low-fat protein like chicken or fish. Then add a bit of monounsaturated fat, like a little olive oil or a few slivered almonds. Do this at every meal and snack, and, presto, you're pretty close to being in the Zone for the next four to six hours. And during that four- to six-hour period, you will be thinking better, performing better, and losing stored body fat—all without hunger. This book will teach you how.

Once you understand what the Zone is and how it works, you will also understand that virtually every dietary recommendation made by the U.S. government and leading nutritional experts is hormonally dead wrong. What is their recommendation? Eat a high-carbohydrate diet. Unfortunately, these authorities seem to have forgotten that the best way to fatten cattle is to feed them excessive amounts of low-fat grain. The best way to fatten humans is also to feed them excessive amounts of low-fat grain, in the form of pasta and bagels. Another popular dietary slogan these days says, "If no fat touches my lips, then no fat reaches my hips." But that is simply not true. Our war on dietary fat really began in earnest fifteen years ago as fat phobia became the norm. And the results are now clear: Americans have become more obese than anyone on the face of the earth.

Obviously, fat was not the enemy. If fat isn't the enemy, then what is? The answer is insulin. It's excess insulin that makes you fat and keeps you fat. And your body produces excessive amounts of insulin when you eat either (1) too many fat-free carbohydrates, or (2) too many calories at a meal. Therefore, when I talk about the Zone, it is really a zone of insulin. Not too high, not too low: a zone of insulin controlled by your diet.

To eat in the Zone is to treat food with the same respect you would give a prescription drug. However, this doesn't mean food must taste like a drug. On the contrary, Zone cooking allows for great-tasting food packed with maximum nutrition. Mastering the Zone is a recipe for lifelong hormonal control, a recipe that pretty much lets you forget about counting calories or grams of fat.

Throughout this book, I will refer to my program as the Zone Diet. Most people think of a diet as a limited time they live in a state of deprivation that allows them to return to old eating habits. The Zone Diet is neither deprivation nor short-term. It is not deprivation because while you're in the Zone, you maintain peak mental and physical performance while consuming the foods you like to eat. And being in the Zone is a lifetime habit, not a short-term fad. The hormonal responses generated by food that allow you to reach the Zone haven't changed for the past 100,000 years, and they are not going to change in your lifetime.

Like any lifestyle change, getting into the Zone takes patience and practice. But within two weeks, if not sooner, you will begin to see a dramatic change in your life. Carbohydrate cravings will be gone, mental focus will be increased, physical performance will be enhanced, and you will lose excess body fat at the fastest possible rate. And you will be well on your way to achieving SuperHealth. That's the kind of lifestyle change anyone should be happy to swallow.

This book is divided into three basic parts. The first describes how to determine your unique protein and carbohydrate requirements and how they work together to form your hormonal carburetor. The second part deals with the construction of balanced Zone meals and contains more than one hundred and fifty new Zone recipes. The final part provides helpful hints that will allow you to stay in the Zone for a lifetime.

If SuperHealth is what you want to achieve, then reaching the Zone and staying there is the way to make it happen. Your grandmother knew this intuitively. Treat this book as a personal user's guide and achieve a precision never imagined by your grandmother. And once you're in the Zone, why would you ever want to leave?

2

YOUR PROTEIN PRESCRIPTION: THE FIRST STEP TO THE ZONE

You're nearly ready to travel toward the Zone, but just as with any trip, some preparation is necessary before you begin the journey. As I said in the first chapter, reaching the Zone is all about insulin control. If you have read *The Zone,* you know that the most important step needed to control insulin is fulfilling your body's unique protein requirements.

Why is protein so important? First, your body requires incoming protein on a continual basis to repair and maintain its critical systems. Your muscles, your immune system, and every enzyme in your body are composed of protein. Every day your body loses protein constantly. Without adequate incoming dietary protein, these critical body functions begin to run down.

But more important, protein is so vital because it stimulates the hormone glucagon. Glucagon has the opposite physiological action to insulin. In fact, glucagon acts as the major governor of excessive insulin production. It is excess insulin that makes you fat, makes you hungry, makes you mentally foggy, decreases your physical performance, and increases the likelihood of chronic disease.

If your goal is to enter the Zone and stay there, then you have to control insulin production, and to do that, protein is the key.

So how much protein should you eat at a meal? Here is the simple answer and handy rule of thumb: **Never consume more low-fat protein in one sitting than you can fit on the palm of your hand.** This means the maximum amount of protein you should eat at a meal is approximately 5 ounces of skinless chicken breast or its equivalent.

Of course, your protein requirement is unique to you and no one else. One size does not fit all. So can you be even more precise about exactly how much protein you need?

The answer is yes, and to make it very easy for you to actually apply, use, and remember just how much protein you need, I have created a nutritional measurement that I call a block. I don't care if you have a Ph.D. in nuclear physics, you probably don't want to have to calculate how many grams of protein you need each day, let alone each meal. But you can apply the block method to any source of protein, be it tofu, tuna, or a steak filet. Your stomach breaks all of them down into simple amino acids for absorption.

My blocks all contain 7 grams of protein. There, I've done the gram counting for you. Now any source of protein is on the same level in terms of amino acid content. Differences in protein density are eliminated. All you have to do is refer to a few simple measurements. One block of protein could be 1 ounce of meat, such as sliced turkey, chicken, or beef. One block of protein could be 1½ ounces of fish, or two egg whites, or ¼ cup of cottage cheese, or 3 ounces of extra-firm tofu. It's all equal to your body. One practical reason I like using blocks is so you can measure the amount of protein you need at each meal on the fingers of one hand.

In Appendix B you will find most of the protein sources (including vegetarian sources) you normally eat, in their appropriate block sizes. With a little practice you'll find that your eyeball becomes a very good judge of protein block size.

Using blocks, you now have a more precise way to determine how much protein is in the food you eat. You can also use blocks to tell you how much protein you need at each meal. **If you are a typical American female, you will need between two and three blocks of protein at every meal, and if you are the typical American male, you will need between three and four blocks of protein at every meal.** This amount of protein is adequate to maintain your muscles and your immune system, but won't exceed your daily requirements.

What if you want even greater precision? First, you have to determine your percent body fat by using the worksheet in

Appendix C. From that you can determine your lean body mass. And from your lean body mass you can begin to figure out exactly how much protein you need every day.

What is lean body mass? You can view your body as consisting of two components. The first is your total fat mass. The other component of your total weight is everything else. This "everything else" component is known as lean body mass. Lean body mass consists of water, muscle, bones, tendons, etc. Your body requires adequate levels of protein to maintain this amount of lean body mass. Obviously, your fat mass doesn't require any incoming dietary protein to maintain it.

Determining your total fat mass can be a downright scary proposition, but you have to do it to establish your starting point. Simply multiply your total weight by your percent body fat. For example, if you weigh 160 pounds and have 25 percent body fat, then your total fat mass will be

$$160 \times 0.25 = 40 \text{ pounds}$$

This means that 40 pounds of pure fat is sitting on your body. Since fat contains 3,500 calories per pound, this means you have approximately 140,000 calories of stored useable fat energy, and this stored energy is the equivalent of the calories in more than 2,000 pancakes!

So to continue the example, if you have 40 pounds of total fat, then what is your lean body mass? Simply subtract your total fat mass (40 pounds) from your total weight (160 pounds). As I said, your fat mass doesn't require any protein to maintain it, only your lean body mass does. So if you weigh 160 pounds and subtract 40 pounds of fat, what is left behind is 120 pounds of lean body mass. This measure gives you half of your Protein Prescription.

The other half of your Protein Prescription is determined by how active you are. Do you primarily watch TV all day (and that includes looking at computer screens all day at work), or are you a world-class athlete working out twice a day? Obviously, the more active you are, the more protein you will need. So we run a continuum from purely sedentary individuals (who only need 0.5 grams of protein per pound of lean body mass per day) to elite athletes (who require double that amount, or 1.0 grams of protein per pound of lean body mass per day). Between those extremes will be your activity level.

To calculate your protein requirements, multiply your lean body mass by your physical activity factor (see below). Now we're finally ready to determine your Protein Prescription: the actual amount of protein that you will require to maintain your lean body mass. Just multiply your lean body mass by your activity factor.

Protein Prescription = Lean Body Mass x Activity Factor

Continuing our example, if you had 120 pounds of lean body mass and were sedentary, you would require 60 grams of protein per day (120 pounds of lean body mass x 0.5 grams of protein/pound of lean body mass). Now divide that 60 grams of protein by 7 grams of protein per block, and you see that you would require about nine protein blocks per day. On the other hand, if you were an elite athlete with 120 pounds of lean body mass, you would require 120 grams of protein per day (120 pounds of lean body mass x 1.0 grams of protein per pound of lean body mass). Divide that 120 grams of protein by 7 grams of protein per block, and you see that you would require about seventeen protein blocks per day. Note that the number of protein blocks required each day to maintain your lean body mass doesn't depend on your gender, only on your lean body mass and physical activity factor.

Listed below are levels of activity in terms of total weekly exercise so you can determine your own protein requirements.

PHYSICAL ACTIVITY FACTOR	GRAMS OF PROTEIN PER POUND OF LEAN BODY MASS
Sedentary	0.5
Light activity (e.g., walking)	0.6
Moderate activity (1.5 hours per week)	0.7
Active (1.5 to 2.5 hours per week)	0.8
Very active (greater than 2.5 hours per week)	0.9
Elite athlete (or weight training five times per week)	1.0

Keep in mind that people tend to overestimate their physical activity, just as they underestimate how much they actually eat. So here are some guidelines. If you walk 30 minutes a day seven times a week, then consider this light activity. If you work out three days a week for about 30 minutes a day, this would constitute moderate activity (this is about 1.5 hours per week of formal exercise). If you are working out five times a week for about 30 minutes (or about 2.5 hours per week), consider yourself active. If you do weight training at least three times a week in addition to working out for more than 2.5 hours per week, you are in the very active category. And finally, if you work out intensely twice a day, consider yourself an elite athlete.

Here is another key Zone rule: **Never consume any more protein than your body needs to maintain your lean body mass, but never eat less. Eating too little is to subject yourself to protein malnutrition.** In other words, stay in balance.

Now that you have your Protein Prescription, treat it like a prescription for a drug. First, you're going to have to take fairly equal doses throughout the day. If you were taking a hypertensive drug, you wouldn't take 5 mg in the morning, 500 mg at noon, and 250 mg at the evening. At least I hope not. More likely you would take three equal doses to maintain blood levels throughout the day and to maintain a therapeutic zone for the drug. Your Protein Prescription is the same. You're going to spread it throughout the day into three meals and two snacks, just like a prescription drug. In Chapter 6, I will show you how to do just that.

Remember, I am not talking about consuming a lot of protein at any one time. The human body can handle only relatively small amounts of protein at a meal. That amount of protein is a maximum of only about 35 grams (about 5 ounces) of low-fat protein per meal. That amount is about the amount you can fit onto the palm of your hand (remember the first quick Zone rule on protein). Or, now that you know about blocks, you can say that it's five blocks of protein. On the Zone Diet, that amount of protein (even for Olympic athletes) should never be exceeded at any meal. By eating small amounts of protein throughout the day, you are spreading your protein requirement evenly into your body, as if you are using an intravenous drip.

This is not to say you have to eat animal protein to be on the

Zone Diet. On the contrary, there are several great vegetarian sources of protein that you can use on this program. One of the best is firm or extra-firm tofu. Most of the carbohydrate has been fermented out of this type of tofu, making it very protein-rich. (Soft tofu, on the other hand, has not been fermented as much and is much richer in carbohydrate.) In many ways, firm and extra-firm tofu are the vegetarian equivalent of cottage cheese.

Unfortunately, tofu is not very protein-dense, so you have to use a lot (about 3 ounces) to get a block of protein. However, some of the inherent limitations of tofu have been overcome by a new generation of soybean-based imitation meat products that actually taste pretty good. Soybean hamburgers, hot dogs, sausages, etc., are all interesting sources of protein that can provide appropriate levels of protein in a vegetarian diet. Taking this one step further, there is also a new generation of soybean protein powders called soybean protein isolates that are not only very protein-dense but also contain a complete spectrum of amino acids (long one of the criticisms of soybean as a protein source). Adding protein powder to a meal (like stirring it into oatmeal in the morning) can be another great way to improve the hormonal balance of a purely vegetarian menu.

What about other traditional vegetarian sources of protein? Unfortunately, they carry either massive amounts of carbohydrate with them (like beans), or they are not very protein-dense (like broccoli). Furthermore, the high fiber content in such vegetarian sources prevents a significant amount of the protein from being digested. Rather than having to make all these correction factors, just make life easier for yourself and treat beans, broccoli, and other vegetable sources as excellent forms of carbohydrates and forget their protein content.

Knowing how much protein you need is only the first step toward the Zone. A Zone Diet is not a high-protein diet, it is a protein-adequate diet. But to have the Zone Diet work correctly you actually have to consume slightly *more* carbohydrate than protein. And like protein, there are limits on carbohydrate consumption: not too much nor too little. Just *how* much is a question that begs to be answered.

3

CARBOHYDRATES: MANNA FROM HEAVEN?

We are led to believe that carbohydrates are the closest thing to manna from heaven. After all, carbohydrates are fat-free. Just as Americans have become obsessive about fat-free foods, they have simultaneously embraced the idea that eating carbohydrates is next to godliness.

You're told that if you are an athlete, eating them will make you run faster. If you are a cardiovascular patient, they will make you well. If you are fat, eating them will make you thin. Sound familiar? It should, because virtually every nutritional publication in this country espouses the moral superiority of carbohydrates to any food that contains fat, and that includes protein.

Yet many of those millions of Americans who have worshipped at the altar of carbohydrates for the past fifteen years show an amazing degree of ignorance about what carbohydrates actually are. Ask most people, and they will tell you that carbohydrates are pasta, bagels, or sweets. If you look them in the eye and ask them what a fruit or vegetable is, they'll usually respond by telling you it's a fruit or it's a vegetable as if those foods are some unique species just recently discovered in the Amazon rain forest. In fact, fruits and vegetables are also carbohydrates.

As I stated in *The Zone*, people are genetically designed to eat primarily fruits and vegetables as their major source of carbohydrates. Grains as a reliable source of food simply did not exist 10,000 years ago. Consequently, the great majority of individuals have still not genetically adapted to eating high-density forms of carbohydrates, such as grains, starches, bread, and pasta.

Carbohydrates act as powerful drugs, a fact that most people just don't realize. As with any drug, excessive intake will cause side effects. In this case, excessive carbohydrate consumption causes your body to overproduce insulin. And too much insulin can make you fat and sluggish, and it can be dangerous.

Excess insulin acts like a loose cannon on the deck of a ship. Elevated insulin induces foggy thinking by reducing blood sugar levels to the brain (think of how hard it is to concentrate three hours after having eaten a big pasta lunch). Elevated insulin will decrease your overall physical performance. Most important, the biochemical effects from elevated insulin will profoundly affect your health. In fact, elevated insulin is the primary predictor of whether you will have a heart attack.

All that said, I want to make it clear that I am not anti-carbohydrate, but I am pro-balance and pro-moderation with respect to carbohydrates and their effect on insulin. Everyone needs to be keenly aware of the effect of carbohydrates on insulin.

If this sounds like carbohydrate-bashing, then let's go back into history and ask just how good carbohydrates were for ancient civilizations. Before the beginning of agriculture 10,000 years ago, people survived very well by eating low-fat protein and fruits and vegetables. This was the diet of most hunter-gatherer societies. It was only with the beginning of agriculture that people made the corresponding switch to a grain-based diet.

Not surprisingly, many diseases of "modern civilization" appeared during this switch to a grain-based diet. How do we know? The mummies tell us. Ancient Egyptian religion placed a great emphasis on preserving the body of the deceased for the afterlife through mummification. Furthermore, mummification was common in all social classes. What was religion then provides a powerful scientific tool now as mummies give us an excellent physical sampling of ancient Egyptian society.

Ancient Egyptians were the first society to follow a diet similar to the one recommended by the guidelines in the new U.S. food pyramid. They ate lots of bread, some vegetables and fruits, and small amounts of meat in the form of fish and waterfowl, and their only fat came from olives. If there was ever an ideal society to study the effects of a high-carbohydrate, low-fat diet, it would be the ancient Egyptians.

What do the mummies have to tell us? A lot of bad news is found under those wraps. First, many of the diseases that we assume appeared only with the advent of modern civilization were in full bloom in the ancient Egyptian society. Tooth decay is one. Although the Egyptians ate no refined sugar, they suffered from terrible tooth decay. This isn't all that surprising when you realize that chewing bread long enough will release a massive amount of sugar into the mouth.

If you want to do a simple experiment, purchase some diagnostic strips that diabetics use to test sugar in their urine. When these sticks turn blue, a significant amount of sugar is present. Now take a piece of bread and chew it for a few minutes in your mouth. Then place the diabetic sugar strip in your mouth and, presto, the strip turns blue. The enzymes in your mouth are turning the bread into pure sugar. It's not so surprising that the Egyptians had such a high degree of tooth decay. This simple experiment also gives you a good idea of how much sugar rushes into your system after you have eaten a piece of bread or a big pasta meal.

Tooth decay is one thing. What about heart disease? The ancient Egyptian diet is similar to the diet recommended by doctors in the United States today to prevent heart disease. You would think that there should be no trace of heart disease in mummies. Wrong.

Analysis of dissected arteries from mummies indicates extensive signs of advanced heart disease. In fact there are estimates that the extent of heart disease in ancient Egypt wasn't all that different from that in present-day America. Furthermore, the medical texts of ancient Egypt, written nearly 3,500 years ago, leave a clear impression that heart disease was widespread. In those texts are descriptions of the symptoms of a heart attack that could have been written yesterday by the American Heart Association. And if that isn't enough, remember the average age of death in ancient Egypt was far younger than it is today, which means heart disease appeared to be rampant in a much younger population.

Finally, what about obesity? Following the ancient Egyptian diet, it would be virtually impossible for anyone to be fat, right? Wrong again. The excess skin flaps in the midsections of mummies indicate extensive obesity in the ancient Egyptians. Of course, no one has ever seen a fat Egyptian in hieroglyphics. Why? Probably for the same reason that anthropologists 2,000 years from now will never see a fat American female in an unearthed copy of *Cosmopolitan* or *Vogue.* Excess body fat simply didn't play well in ancient Egypt, just as it doesn't play well in present-day America.

As philosopher George Santayana said, "Those who don't learn from history are condemned to repeat it." The Egyptian mummies are history, and it appears that the American public is repeating their fate.

You don't have to rely on the study of ancient Egyptians to come to the same conclusion about excess consumption of grains or starches. For example, a study published in 1996 in *Lancet* demonstrated that Italians who consumed the highest levels of pasta had the highest levels of breast cancer. But nowhere did anyone see a headline in any leading newspaper stating that pasta increases the risk of breast cancer. Obviously, pasta-bashing is politically incorrect.

Furthermore, two other studies from the same research group in Italy indicate that excessive pasta consumption is also linked to increases in colon cancer and stomach cancer. On the other hand, every major study has indicated that people who increased their consumption of fruits and vegetables had reduced rates of cancer and heart disease.

All this leads to the quick Zone rule on carbohydrates: **Let most of your carbohydrates come from fruits and vegetables, and use grains, starches, pasta, and bread in moderation.** In Table 3–1, carbohydrates are divided into two classes: favorable and unfavorable.

Table 3.1
Carbohydrate Quick List

FAVORABLE	UNFAVORABLE
Fruits	Starches (potatoes, rice, etc.)
Vegetables	Grains (cereals, pasta, bread, etc.)

Now eating more fruits and vegetables and fewer grains, starches, and pasta is a good way to begin heading toward the Zone. But can you become even more precise in controlling insulin? The answer is definitely yes. To start, you'll need a consistent measurement of the amount of carbohydrate in the foods you eat to determine their ability to stimulate insulin secretion. This could be done by measuring calories or grams, but there is a much easier way. Simply apply the block method to carbohydrates. When you redefine carbohydrates into blocks, it becomes very easy to get precisely into the Zone.

Some carbohydrates, such as fruits and vegetables, are not very carbohydrate-dense. In other words you have to eat a lot of them to get the same amount of carbohydrate found in very carbohydrate-dense sources, such as grains, starches, and pasta. By using carbohydrate blocks, you have a simple way to measure the amount of carbohydrate you need to eat, despite different densities of carbohydrates from various sources.

That is true even with the complicating factor of the fiber content of carbohydrates. The amount of insulin your body will produce is based on only the amount of carbohydrate that actually enters into the bloodstream as the simple sugar glucose. Fiber doesn't count. Therefore, when calculating carbohydrate blocks, you subtract the fiber to end up with the actual amount of carbohydrate that actually enters the bloodstream.

And it is only the carbohydrate that actually enters the bloodstream, the *insulin-promoting* carbohydrate, that I count to construct my easy-to-use carbohydrate blocks. For example, 1½ cups of broccoli has the same amount of insulin-promoting carbohydrate as ¼ cup of cooked pasta. Anyone can eat 1 cup of cooked pasta, but eating 6 cups of cooked broccoli is pretty hard work! Yet they both contain the same amount of insulin-promoting carbohydrate. Since the Zone Diet recommends eating primarily fruits and vegetables for its carbohydrate sources, it is a diet that is exceptionally rich in fiber, yet moderate in the amount of insulin-promoting carbohydrates consumed.

Ultimately, all carbohydrate blocks contain 9 grams of insulin-promoting carbohydrate. Why 9 grams? Because 9 grams of insulin-promoting carbohydrate is the exact amount you need to eat to hormonally balance the 7 grams of protein in my definition of a protein block. Now all you have to do is keep the amount of protein blocks equal to the number of carbohydrate blocks at any meal. And you will have an exceptionally easy way to construct Zone meals, as I will show in later chapters.

You can also appreciate that eating most of your carbohydrates from fruits and vegetables will supply not only large amounts of fiber, but also very significant levels of vitamins and minerals for a given amount of insulin-promoting carbohydrate. On the other hand, high-density carbohydrates such as grains, starches, and pasta supply relatively little fiber, vitamins, and minerals for the same given amount of insulin-promoting carbohydrate. I have illustrated this in Table 3-2, which compares the fiber, vitamin, and mineral content of different types of carbohydrate containing the same amount of insulin-promoting carbohydrate.

Table 3-2
Comparison of Fiber, Vitamin, and Mineral Content of Different Carbohydrates Containing One Block of Insulin-Promoting Carbohydrate

CARBOHYDRATE TYPE	FIBER	VITAMIN C	MAGNESIUM	CALCIUM
Favorable				
Broccoli (1½ cups)	3.6 g	55 mg	27 mg	104 mg
Red Pepper (3 peppers)	3.6 g	423 mg	21 mg	21 mg
Strawberries (1 cup)	1.9 g	91 mg	34 mg	45 mg
Orange (½)	1.6 g	40 mg	7 mg	25 mg
Unfavorable				
Pasta (2 ounces dry)	0.3 g	0.5 mg	6 mg	2.5 mg
White Rice (½ ounce dry)	0.1 g	0.0 mg	4 mg	1 mg

It doesn't take a rocket scientist to figure out that you will obtain a lot more fiber, vitamins, and minerals eating favorable carbohydrates (fruits and vegetables) than by eating unfavorable carbohydrates (grains, starches, and pasta). In fact, it's hard to understand why any nutritionist would recommend large amounts of pasta or rice as the base of any healthy diet.

One added complicating factor for carbohydrates is the glycemic index. The higher the glycemic index of a carbohydrate, the faster it enters the bloodstream as sugar. You may have been told in health class that all carbohydrates are either simple or complex. Well, they are in the mouth, but not in your stomach. All carbohydrates, whether simple or complex, have to be broken down into simple sugars before being absorbed by the body and entering the bloodstream. But it was only in 1980 that anyone bothered to ask the seemingly obvious question: "How fast does any carbohydrate actually get into the bloodstream?" The answer is exceedingly important if you're a Type II diabetic. (Indeed, 95 percent of all diabetics are Type II diabetics. They actually make too much insulin, and that's why virtually all of them are overweight.) The answer is also important if you are overweight, as high levels of insulin prevent the use of your stored body fat.

The only simple sugar that can actually enter the bloodstream is glucose, and the faster glucose appears in the bloodstream, the more insulin you make. Therefore, carbohydrates with a high glycemic index will have a greater effect on insulin secretion compared to carbohydrates with a lower glycemic index. The more insulin you make, the worse your diabetic condition becomes if you're a Type II diabetic (or the fatter you become if you happen to be overweight).

You might think that simple carbohydrates would enter the bloodstream faster than complex carbohydrates. When the first experiments were done at the University of Toronto, this often wasn't the case.

Some simple carbohydrates, such as table sugar, enter the bloodstream more slowly than more seemingly dietetically correct breakfast cereals, such as cornflakes. In other cases, it was found that the sugar in ice cream was entering the bloodstream far more slowly than complex carbohydrates found in a bagel. What was going on? It turns out that a lot of things were.

First, let's look at table sugar. Table sugar is composed of half glucose and half fructose, which is quickly broken down into both simple sugars. The glucose half is rapidly absorbed and enters the bloodstream quickly because it is already in the form your body can use. Fructose, although rapidly absorbed, has to be converted into glucose in the liver before it enters the bloodstream in the use-able form of glucose. And this is a very slow process. The end result is that the overall rise of blood glucose is retarded. Since fruits primarily contain fructose, they have a very low glycemic index and stimulate insulin production far less than other carbohy-drates, such as grains or starches.

For instance, the long-considered dietetically correct breakfast cereal is essentially pure glucose linked by chemical bonds. These bonds are very easily broken in the stomach, allowing glucose to rush into the bloodstream at a faster rate than the carbohydrate from table sugar. Therefore, it is time to rethink what is simple and what is complex.

Then consider ice cream, which also has a low glycemic index. The fat in the ice cream acts like a control rod, slowing the entry of any car-bohydrates into the bloodstream. That's why the sugar in ice cream enters the bloodstream at a much slower rate than the glucose in a bagel.

Fiber can also play a role in determining the glycemic index, but not all fiber. There are two types of fiber, soluble and insoluble. Insoluble fiber includes such things as cellulose and bran, whereas soluble fiber includes such things as pectin, which is found in apples. (Remember what your grandmother said about an apple a day.) Soluble fiber represents another type of control rod that slows the rate of entry of any carbohydrate into the bloodstream. The type of fiber you find in a breakfast cereal is insoluble fiber, which has virtually no effect on carbohydrate entry.

Finally, how you cook a carbohydrate will also have a large effect on its glycemic index. The more you cook or process a car-bohydrate, the more you break down its cell structure, allowing faster digestion. This is why refried beans have a much higher glycemic index than slightly cooked kidney beans. And when you go to convenience carbohydrates such as instant potatoes and instant rice, the glycemic index is dramatically increased. Obviously you pay a hormonal price for convenience.

And the food with perhaps the highest glycemic index on record? It's those puffed rice cakes, which have become the staple of every dieter on a high-carbohydrate, low-fat program.

Finally, let me say a word about alcohol. For all intents and purposes, the body treats alcohol as if it were a carbohydrate. As a result, any alcohol consumption has to be treated as if you were consuming carbohydrates, and each type of alcohol (wine, beer, or distilled spirits) represents a different carbohydrate block amount (found in Appendix B).

Here's another Zone rule on carbohydrates: Primarily use carbohydrates that are both low-density (thereby providing maximum fiber, vitamins, and minerals) and low-glycemic (so carbohydrates enter the blood at a slow and controlled rate). Conversely, unfavorable carbohydrates are high-density and high-glycemic carbohydrates. This is not to say you can never eat unfavorable carbohydrates, but they should be used with greater moderation, probably no more than a quarter of your total carbohydrate blocks, especially if you are genetically prone to being insulin-sensitive to carbohydrates.

How can you tell your degree of insulin sensitivity to carbohydrates without complicated medical testing? Simply eat a big pasta meal at lunch. If you begin falling asleep by three o'clock in the afternoon, then you are definitely insulin sensitive to carbohydrates.

Bear in mind that being insulin sensitive is very different from having constantly elevated levels of insulin (this is called hyperinsulinemia). When you are hyperinsulinemic, you are fast-tracking yourself to a heart attack. If you have an existing heart condition, you are also probably hyperinsulinemic, and it is likely that you come from that genetic pool of individuals who are genetically prone to producing high levels of insulin in response to any carbohydrate.

Now, of course, your body does need a constant intake of carbohydrate for optimal brain function. Too little carbohydrate in the bloodstream, and your brain will not function efficiently. Too much carbohydrate in the bloodstream, and your body responds by increasing the secretion of insulin to drive down blood sugar to a level too low to allow your brain to function effectively.

What your body needs is a zone of incoming carbohydrate. Not too much, not too little, just like protein. This maintains a zone of insulin. As I have said before, elevated insulin is the reason you get fat and stay fat.

But just how does excess carbohydrate consumption and corresponding insulin secretion increase your body fat? As I said in *The Zone,* insulin is your body's storage and locking hormone. The elevated insulin levels generated from a large carbohydrate meal prevent your body from using any of its stored fat for energy. In other words, it prevents you from burning the fat you already have.

Not only that, but humans can store unlimited amounts of excess calories as fat, and insulin is the key trigger. A unique evolutionary mechanism has evolved to limit our immediate use of incoming dietary fat for energy when excess carbohydrates are available in the bloodstream. Since incoming dietary fat is not used immediately for energy, the elevated presence of insulin (due to higher carbohydrate intake) ensures that the incoming dietary fat is driven into the adipose tissue for future storage: a clever but insidious process in the land where carbohydrate is king. This same evolutionary process is the reason that the combination of fat and excess carbohydrates (like a potato with butter) in a meal can be such an accelerator for fat accumulation.

Fear not. By now you have the beginnings of some very powerful dietary tools (protein, fat, and fiber) to work to decrease insulin secretion caused by carbohydrates. Protein stimulates glucagon, which reduces insulin secretion, and fat and fiber slow down the rate of entry of any carbohydrate to further reduce insulin secretion. Use these tools wisely.

Here is a summary of some simple Zone rules on carbohydrate.

1. Eat primarily low-density carbohydrates, like fruits and most fiber-rich vegetables.
2. Make sure that you consume primarily carbohydrates that have a low glycemic index.
3. Keep track of the total number of carbohydrate blocks that you are consuming in a given meal. By eating low-density carbohydrates, it is very easy to avoid overconsumption of carbohydrate blocks.

And the amount of carbohydrate you need to consume to maintain insulin in a tight zone? That is determined by the amount of protein you require at the same meal. This is the essence of the Zone Diet, the balance of protein and carbohydrates at every meal.

However, you need one last critical ingredient. The most dreaded three-letter word in America: FAT.

4

IT TAKES FAT TO BURN FAT

You're not dreaming. As ironic as it sounds, it does take fat to burn fat. But for this seemingly paradoxical statement to have meaning, you have to be thinking hormonally, not calorically.

How can fat be such an ally in burning your own stored body fat? I'll give you the reasons. First, incoming dietary fat has no effect on insulin. Carbohydrate is the major stimulator of insulin, and even protein can have a slight stimulatory effect on insulin, but fat is a big zero when it comes to insulin stimulation. So eating fat will not cause your body to store more fat.

Second, fat slows down the entry of carbohydrates into the bloodstream. In essence, fat acts like a control rod in a nuclear reactor to prevent an overproduction of insulin. The slower the rate that carbohydrates enter the bloodstream, the lower the insulin production. And the lower the insulin levels, the more likely you are to release stored body fat for energy. So in fact, fat is really your ally in chipping away stored body fat.

Third, fat causes the release of the hormone cholecystokinin (CCK) from the stomach. CCK goes directly to the brain to say, "Stop eating." So in essence, fat is your primary hormonal off-switch for eating.

Therefore, when you take much of the fat out of your diet and replace it with carbohydrate, you not only rob food of its taste, but you distort the hormonal signals that stop you from overconsuming calories, and *increase* your likelihood of storing fat by increasing insulin levels.

I'm not advocating fat gluttony, just recommending that you add enough additional fat to your diet to help your body reduce insulin secretion.

For although fat has no direct effect on insulin, you do want to keep your intake of saturated fat low (but again probably not for the reasons that you might expect). All the membranes in your body operate best in a zone of fluidity. If membranes are too fluid, they don't provide the rigidity required for proper function. They begin to look like a Salvador Dali watch. The body recognizes this fact and will make enough saturated fat to increase the viscosity of the membrane to maintain the necessary fluidity zone even if you are eating no saturated fat at all. On the other hand, if you are eating a lot of saturated fat, the cell membranes become too rigid, and resemble molasses in winter. Since the body has no mechanism to make polyunsaturated fat, it is unable to improve the fluidity of the membrane. In this rigid membrane environment, your body's receptors (especially the insulin receptor) don't function very well, and the body has to pump out more insulin to bring down blood sugar levels. This leads to insulin resistance and eventually hyperinsulinemia. Therefore, it simply makes good sense to keep your saturated fat intake to a minimum.

While reducing saturated fat is strongly recommended, it doesn't mean throwing the baby out with the bathwater. You do need a constant intake of *polyunsaturated* fats, which are the building blocks of eicosanoids.

What are eicosanoids? Simply stated, they are the most powerful hormones in your body. They control every cell, every organ, every system. Only a handful of physicians know about them, let alone the general public. This is because these hormones are extremely short-lived, never travel through the bloodstream, and are all but invisible to scientific study. Yet in a sense they are the molecular glue that holds your body together, and that's why the 1982 Nobel Prize in medicine was awarded for research, which underscores just how important these hormones are.

Eicosanoids are the hormones that will dictate whether you suffer a heart attack, how well you can rally your immune system, whether you have pain or inflammation, plus a myriad of other controlling functions. Yet as with all hormonal systems, their function is a matter of balance. If you have read *The Zone,* you know there are both "good" and "bad" eicosanoids, and you require a balance of both types to maintain SuperHealth. In essence, you want to maintain an eicosanoid zone.

And what can destroy that delicate balance of eicosanoids? An overproduction of insulin. This is why maintaining relatively constant levels of insulin is so important to the Zone Diet. Excessive levels of insulin cause a corresponding overproduction of one particular polyunsaturated fatty acid called arachidonic acid.

Your body needs some arachidonic acid because you will always need some amount of bad eicosanoids to maintain that hormonal balance. However, excessive levels of this fatty acid may be one of the most dangerous events you will ever encounter. Many chronic disease conditions (heart disease, cancer, diabetes, arthritis, etc.) are a consequence of elevated levels of bad eicosanoids derived from arachidonic acid. If you inject a rabbit with high amounts of arachidonic acid, it will be dead within minutes.

And where do you find excessive levels of arachidonic acid? In fatty red meats, egg yolks, and organ meats. Just as you should avoid saturated fats, you should also keep these dietary sources of fat that are rich in arachidonic acid to a minimum.

But simply avoiding dietary sources rich in arachidonic acid is not enough. You should also avoid consuming too much of another kind of polyunsaturated fat, known as omega–6 essential fatty acids. With excessive intake of this type of polyunsaturated fat, you run another risk, as you can potentially begin to overload your system and force it into making too many "bad" eicosanoids and create a hormonal cascade that can hugely undermine your efforts to achieve SuperHealth (see Chapters 4 and 12 on eicosanoids in *The Zone*). This is because excessive levels of omega–6 fatty acids (especially if coupled with high levels of insulin) can eventually increase the levels of arachidonic acid.

What are common sources rich in omega–6 fatty acids? Primarily oils like sunflower, safflower, and soybean. Since you will get all the omega–6 essential fatty acids you need by eating adequate levels of low-fat protein, you want to limit any added dietary fat sources rich in omega–6 fatty acids.

What your body really needs are adequate amounts of another kind of polyunsaturated fats, called omega–3 fatty acids, particularly the most important fatty acid in this family, eicosapentaenoic acid (EPA). EPA helps your body avoid the same negative hormonal cascade that excess intakes of omega–6 fatty acids can trigger. If you are keeping your intake of omega–6 fatty acids low, then you won't need that much EPA (probably only 200–400 mg per day). The best source of EPA is fish (with salmon the richest). Eating adequate amounts of EPA should be a primary dietary goal. If you don't like fish you can always get some EPA in your diet the same way your grandmother did: by taking cod liver oil.

If you are restricting the amounts of saturated fat and arachidonic acid, moderating the amounts of omega–6 polyunsaturated fats, and taking in relatively limited amounts of omega–3 essential fatty acids like EPA, then what type of fat should you eat to help yourself burn fat? The answer is monounsaturated fat. It's a hormonally neutral fat. It has no adverse effect on membrane fluidity. It has no effect on eicosanoids, it's easy to find, and it tastes great. Excellent sources of monounsaturated fat are olives, avocado (especially in the form of guacamole), and certain nuts such as macadamia, pistachio, cashew, and almond. Of course, you may always use olive oil. Besides, who could find fault in the concept of eating macadamia nuts, almonds, olives, and guacamole to burn excess body fat?

As with protein and carbohydrate blocks, there are also fat blocks. A fat block is only 1.5 grams of fat, which translates into one macadamia nut or ⅓ teaspoon of olive oil. As you can see, this is not a program of fat gluttony, but a method of using controlled amounts of fat to get the maximum tuning of what I call your hormonal carburetor.

And it is learning how to use your hormonal carburetor that is the true key to mastering the Zone.

5

YOUR HORMONAL CARBURETOR

To reach the Zone you must keep insulin in a tight range. Not too high, not too low. It's a lot like the carburetor in your car, which balances the gas and air going to your car's engine. Have you ever tried to run a car all on gas or all on air? You can't do it. You need a combination of both to make the engine run. The better you control that ratio of gas to air, the less wear and tear to the engine and thus the greater the mileage you get from your car.

In principle, your body behaves no differently. You can't run the body on all carbohydrate or all protein. You need a combination of both. You need a hormonal carburetor. Unfortunately, your body doesn't come fully installed. That's where the Zone Diet comes in. It keeps insulin in a tight range and things running smoothly, so that you can extend your own mileage.

Since no two people are alike, the range of effective protein-to-carbohydrate ratios for this human hormonal carburetor will vary, but for everyone it has boundaries. These boundaries are based on the ratio of insulin-promoting carbohydrates to absorbable protein consumed at every meal.

For the vast majority of individuals this carburetor works best at a 1:1 ratio of protein to carbohydrate blocks (this is how the block sizes for protein and carbohydrate were chosen). Nobody's hormonal carburetor ranges very far from that. And in Chapter 7, I will show you how to make any slight adjustments you may need.

But first you have to learn how to maintain this carburetor. As with all science, the more precise you are, the better the results. Still, your eye can provide you with a pretty good indicator of how you are doing in terms of hitting this ratio. Not surprisingly, I call this technique the eyeball method. Not as precise as the block method (described below), the eyeball method is easier to follow, especially when dining out. Just use this simple rule: Whatever the amount of low-fat protein you plan to eat, let that size (and really the volume) determine the amount of carbohydrates you're going to eat at the same time. If the carbohydrates you plan to eat are *unfavorable* carbohydrates (grains, starches, pasta, bagels, etc.), then make their volume equal to the volume of the low-fat protein portion you are going to eat. If you plan to eat *favorable* carbohydrates (fruits and vegetables), then you can double the volume of the low-fat protein portion. This method won't give quite the same precision of hormonal control as the block method, but at least your hormonal carburetor will never be too far out of tune.

Now, let's begin learning about the block method. A 1:1 ratio of protein-to-carbohydrate blocks is the equivalent of 7 grams of protein for every 9 grams of insulin-promoting carbohydrates (a protein-to-carbohydrate ratio of about 0.75). Don't let the math scare you. If you follow the techniques given in this book, hitting these ratios to maintain an ideal hormonal balance will become second nature (as will making the needed adjustments). And one of the most important adjustments is to add fat.

For every protein block and carbohydrate block you consume, you should add one fat block. This is not adding a lot of fat, since one fat block is defined as only 1.5 grams of fat, but this extra fat (especially monounsaturated fat) will be key to maintaining the ideal functioning of your hormonal carburetor. It's like going to a Chinese restaurant. Choose one item from column A (protein blocks), one item from column B (carbohydrate blocks), and one item from column C (fat blocks).

When you finish constructing your meal, the number of protein blocks, carbohydrate blocks, and fat blocks on your plate will be the same. So here is the block rule for constructing Zone meals: Always have equal numbers of protein, carbohydrate, and fat blocks at every meal.

Since a carbohydrate block (9 grams) is larger than a protein block (7 grams), you always consume more carbohydrate than protein at every meal on a Zone Diet. Therefore a Zone Diet can't be called a low-carbohydrate diet. Likewise since people are not consuming excessive amounts of carbohydrates on a Zone Diet, it can't be called a high-carbohydrate diet. I guess the only way to describe a Zone Diet is a carbohydrate-moderate diet. Also, since fat blocks are very low in total fat, the Zone Diet can't be called a high-fat diet. In fact the total amount of fat in a Zone Diet is very low in absolute grams.

Overall moderation is the real key to understanding the Zone. Not too much, not too little. Not too much protein, but not too little. Not too much fat, but not too little. Not too much carbohydrate, but not too little.

Most diets are actually almost formulated to let you be a glutton. High-protein diet advocates say eat all the protein and fat you want, but drastically restrict carbohydrates. High-carbohydrate diet advocates say eat all the carbohydrate you want, but drastically restrict fat. Between both extremes lies the Zone.

Controlling insulin is key to reaching the Zone, but you don't have to give up carbohydrates to achieve this goal as long as you are willing to pay close attention to the ratio of protein and carbohydrate blocks at each meal. In fact, in a recent clinical study done at the University of Geneva in 1996, fat loss in patients following what was essentially a Zone Diet was exactly the same as for the patients following a much more restrictive carbohydrate diet, even though insulin levels were much lower in the highly restrictive carbohydrate diet. This is why the Zone Diet is based more on balance than on elimination. When insulin levels drop too low, many of the negative side effects (fatigue due to electrolyte loss, irritability, constipation, loss of muscle mass, etc.) associated with the high-protein diets of the 1970s become readily apparent. And this is why the constant balance of protein to carbohydrate at every meal is so important in the Zone Diet.

In many ways, I would liken current extreme diets to the early days of birth control pills, when it was thought that massive amounts of hormones were needed to prevent ovulation. Now we know that far smaller amounts do an excellent job. Likewise, the drastic restriction of carbohydrates will decrease insulin, but you don't have to restrict them nearly as much to lose excess body fat if you pay closer attention to your hormonal carburetor, which you now know is controlled by the protein-to-carbohydrate ratio of the meals you eat.

Finally, what about calories? Don't they count? Well, they do and they don't. Let me explain. Caloric thinking says, "A calorie is a calorie," and since a gram of fat has more than twice the calories of a gram of carbohydrate, the fastest way to reduce calorie intake is to drastically reduce dietary fat. But hormonal thinking says, "A calorie of fat has a different hormonal effect than a calorie of protein, which has a still different hormonal effect than a calorie of carbohydrate." So on the Zone Diet, it's not the number of calories on which you should focus. It's their hormonal effects.

This was demonstrated in a classic study by Kekwick and Pawan at the Middlesex Hospital in London nearly forty years ago. Under hospital-ward conditions, various 1,000-calorie-per-day diets were compared to see their effect on weight loss. If weight loss was simply a matter of calories, then regardless of the makeup of the calories, all patients would have experienced the same weight loss. Yet a 1,000-calorie-per-day diet consisting of 90 percent carbohydrates actually caused the patients to gain weight, while they lost weight on all the other 1,000-calorie-per-day diets that had a much lower carbohydrate content.

The hormonal carburetor also takes care of controlling calorie intake for you. Evolution has equipped us with unique hormonal control mechanisms that tell us to stop eating too many calories. The key player in that hormonal stop is called cholecystokinin, or CCK, and fat is the primary stimulator of CCK. As I said in Chapter 4, by reducing the fat in a meal, you are in essence short-circuiting your "stop eating" hormone.

Sound familiar? It probably does if you are on a high-carbohydrate, low-fat, and low-protein diet. Hungry all the time? Don't think you have enough willpower to stop eating so much? You don't need willpower to stop eating calories, you need science. That's what the Zone Diet is all about.

But also bear in mind that this is not an invitation to caloric gluttony. Excessive consumption of too many calories, no matter how well balanced hormonally, will lead to accumulation of excess body fat. But if you stick to your Protein Prescription (outlined in Chapter 2), it will be virtually impossible to consume too many calories on the Zone Diet because of all the hormonal control systems you are putting in play to stop overconsuming total calories.

In fact, the Zone Diet is a low-calorie diet ranging from 1,000 to 1,600 calories a day for most individuals. Should you be concerned about achieving this seemingly low number of calories on a Zone Diet? No, because, paradoxically, the biggest complaint about the Zone Diet is that people can't eat all their food, particularly if they are consuming most of their carbohydrate blocks in the form of favorable carbohydrates (fruits and vegetables with their low carbohydrate densities). To explain this seeming paradox, I have to go into a little more detail.

As I described in *The Zone*, the average American male or female carries at least 100,000 calories of stored body fat at any one time. Put in perspective, this is equivalent to eating 1,700 pancakes. That's a pretty big meal.

The calories you need are already sitting in your body. You just need a hormonal ATM card to release them. That's what your hormonal carburetor can be viewed as, your internal hormonal ATM card that will help you release some of those "fat pancakes" on your body. If you have the right hormonal ATM card, you won't have to eat as many calories to provide your daily caloric requirements. That is because the rest of the calories you need to fulfill your energy needs will come from those "fat pancakes" (having the right ATM card does assume you are in the Zone). On the other hand, if you don't have the correct hormonal ATM card (because you are eating a high-carbohydrate diet), you'll need to take in more incoming calories. And those 1,700 or more "fat pancakes" already on your body will stay there.

That same hormonal ATM card also lets you maintain relatively constant blood sugar levels by releasing stored carbohydrate from the liver. The end result is that you maintain high levels of mental acuity and focus along with a lack of hunger because the brain is now getting all the blood sugar it needs to function optimally. So once you tune up your hormonal carburetor, you will continually access stored body fat, maintain peak mental alertness, and not be hungry for four to six hours after a meal. Does it sound like it's worthwhile to control that carburetor at every meal? I would like to think so, unless you want to be continually mentally sluggish, perform poorly throughout the day, and risk being constantly over-weight.

Obviously, you want to tap into your caloric bank account only until you reach your ideal weight. A good rule of thumb is that your weight as an adult should be what it was at age eighteen. An even better estimation of an ideal body weight comes from the old (i.e., 1959) Metropolitan Life Tables relating size to weight. As Americans have gotten fatter, the recommended weights on such tables have been moved higher, so the older tables actually give better recommendations.

In reality there is no ideal weight, only an ideal percent body fat. That will be 15 percent for males and 22 percent for females. If you have any question about your body fat, simply stand stark naked in front of a mirror. If you're a male and don't have any "love handles," then you're probably close to 15 percent body fat. If you're a female and you have no "cellulite," then you're probably at about 22 percent body fat. Appendix C provides simple tables to determine your percent body fat.

The Zone Diet is designed as if you were already at your ideal percent body fat because at that point you're maintaining your lean body mass while you have used up your extra "fat pancakes." Once you get to your ideal percent body fat, you don't change your diet, because you've been eating as if you were already there from day one. Since the Zone Diet is controlled by your protein require-ments, the only time you ever change your protein intake is when you change your physical activity level or see a significant change in your lean body mass.

Can you achieve even a lower percent body fat? Of course you can, and should. But it's going to take more effort, and that usually means exercise. And is there a lower limit when your body fat can become too low? Certainly. For most males it's about 7 percent and for females about 13 percent. But now we're talking about world-class athletes. Below these levels of body fat, performance suffers. Individuals in this lower range of body fat will need more incoming calories to prevent their percent body fat from falling below a level at which performance will be compromised.

How do these people increase their calories? Will they add more protein to their diet? No, because their protein consumption is already adequate to maintain their lean body mass. Will they add more carbohydrate to their diet? No, because extra carbohydrate will increase insulin and destroy the delicate hormonal carburetor that they are trying to maintain.

What's left? The answer is that they have to add more fat to their diet. That's right, extra fat. This extra fat acts like a caloric ballast to add more calories to their diet and let them maintain a percent body fat in which their performance is optimal. In fact, some of the elite athletes I work with need nearly 60 percent of their calories as fat to maintain peak performance. But for most elite athletes, their fat content on the Zone Diet will be approximately 40–45 percent of total calories. This extra fat should be primarily monounsaturated fat, and should their body fat begin to increase beyond a determined level, they can simply decrease the amount of extra dietary fat they have begun to eat so that their percent body fat remains at the level at which they perform best.

Before you start buying extra jars of macadamia nuts or bottles of olive oil, remember that we are talking about very lean, highly athletic individuals. Here's a good rule of thumb to determine the level of leanness for males. As mentioned earlier, if you don't have any "love handles," then you are about 15 percent body fat. When you can raise your arm and see your ribs, then you have about 13 percent body fat. At about 10 percent body fat you can clearly see your abdominal muscles. If you're a female, simply add another 7 percentage points to the male numbers at each level of leanness, and the same criteria apply. When you can see your abs (for both males and females), then it's time to start adding more fat to your diet.

And this is the only difference between diets designed for Olympic athletes and Type II diabetics. The Olympic athletes will need more protein (because of their greater lean body mass and higher levels of physical activity) and more fat (to maintain their percent body fat in an ideal range). Other than that their meal plans are virtually the same. In Chapter 8, entitled "A Week in the Zone," you will see these diets laid out in more detail.

So how do you construct meals with the ideal block ratio of protein, carbohydrate, and fat to keep insulin in a tight zone like a drug? The next chapter shows you how. Let's spend a day in the Zone.

6

PUTTING IT ALL TOGETHER: A DAY IN THE ZONE

Constructing Zone meals starts with your individual Protein Prescription. Simply take the blocks of protein you require in the course of a day, and spread these blocks throughout the day like a prescription drug. Your daily meal plan is going to consist of three meals per day and two snacks (each snack containing one block).

Another key to the Zone is timing: Never let more than five hours go by without a Zone meal or snack. The body requires food intake on a relatively precise time schedule, just like taking a drug. This timing will maintain the appropriate hormonal levels throughout the day. For example, if you eat breakfast at 7 A.M., then plan to have lunch no later than noon. Since most people eat dinner at 7 P.M., you will have to have a one-block snack at 5 P.M. as a hormonal "touch-up." Finally, you want to have another hormonal touch-up before you go to bed because you are entering an eight-hour cycle of sleep.

I can't emphasize enough how important this late-night snack is because it sets the stage for the correct hormonal environment to facilitate all the repair processes that take place during sleep. In addition, it prevents any nocturnal hypoglycemia, as your brain still requires a supply of energy throughout the night. In fact, the best time to eat is when you're not hungry, which means your blood sugar levels are being maintained. This is just like determining the best time to take hypertensive medications, which is when your blood pressure is still under control.

Once you know your protein block requirements, the only thing you have to remember is the size of the blocks of the protein sources you like to eat. Just memorize these from Appendix B and use your fingers to keep track at each meal. And since your carbohydrate block requirements are exactly the same number as your protein blocks, you can keep track of those on your other hand. Just make sure those blocks are always in balance.

So let's say you are eating four protein blocks at each meal and one block of protein at each snack (a typical amount for an American male). Your meal schedule would look like this:

	BREAKFAST	LUNCH	AFTERNOON SNACK	DINNER	LATE-NIGHT SNACK
Protein Blocks	4	4	1	4	1

Now for every protein block in a meal or snack, plan to add one carbohydrate block. This will make your meal schedule look like this:

	BREAKFAST	LUNCH	AFTERNOON SNACK	DINNER	LATE-NIGHT SNACK
Protein Blocks	4	4	1	4	1
Carbohydrate Blocks	4	4	1	4	1

So far, it seems pretty easy. Now here is the hardest part for most people to grasp. You have to add fat, especially if you want to lose excess body fat. As paradoxical as that sounds, it's true if you understand hormonal thinking. If you really want to control insulin, you always have to add some extra fat to your meals.

But remember you are eating just enough added fat to tune up your hormonal carburetor. Now your meal schedule is finally complete:

	BREAKFAST	LUNCH	AFTERNOON SNACK	DINNER	LATE-NIGHT SNACK
Protein Blocks	4	4	1	4	1
Carbohydrate Blocks	4	4	1	4	1
Fat Blocks	4	4	1	4	1

By reducing everything you eat to precalculated food blocks, you now have a mathematically precise way of adjusting your hormonal carburetor based on the food you like to eat and therefore *will* eat. This is not based on the food someone else hopes you will eat, but the food you actually like to eat today. Everything is now based on your Protein Prescription. And as you can see, constructing Zone meals is actually pretty simple.

To show you how simple it is, let's look at some examples of four blocks of protein, carbohydrate, and fat. Figure 6–1 shows examples of four blocks of most low-fat protein (I threw the bacon in just to give an example of high-fat protein).

Obviously fourteen strips of bacon is not your best possible protein choice, because (1) it's not very dense in protein, and (2) it car-

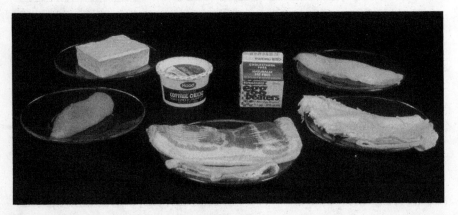

Figure 6-1. Summary of Protein Blocks

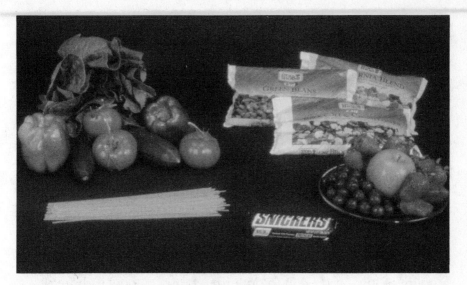

Figure 6-2. Summary of Carbohydrate Blocks

ries a lot of saturated fat, but that is the amount you would require if bacon were your protein choice. The other choices, such as 4 ounces of skinless chicken breast, or 6 ounces of flounder, or 1 cup of egg substitutes, or even 12 ounces of firm tofu, are all better selections. Every one of these choices contains four blocks of protein.

Now that you've chosen your protein for a meal, it's time to choose a carbohydrate that contains four blocks. Possible selections are shown in Figure 6–2.

Obviously, like the bacon, the Snickers bar would not be your best choice, but it does contain four blocks of carbohydrate. If a Snickers bar is not your idea of a great source of carbohydrate, then what about 2 ounces of uncooked pasta? If pasta is your choice, your four blocks doesn't give you much to eat, because 2 ounces would wipe out your carbohydrate allotment for that meal. Could you have made better carbohydrate choices than a Snickers bar or 2 ounces of pasta? Of course. How about the contents of all three bags of the vegetables? Although this would seem like a lot of food (and it is), the high fiber content means that this mass of vegetables contains the same amount of insulin-promoting carbohydrate as the 2 ounces of pasta.

No one in their right mind is going to eat that amount of vegetables, but it does illustrate the differences in insulin-promoting carbohydrate densities of various food sources. Likewise, the other choices (the entire plate of fruit or the massive salad) in Figure 6–2 all contain four blocks of insulin-promoting carbohydrate.

While most people will choose only one protein source per meal, most people will mix and match carbohydrates. Just make sure those carbohydrates don't exceed four blocks. As an example, you could have ¼ cup of cooked pasta, 2 cups of steamed vegetables, and ½ cup of grapes. These are four carbohydrate blocks. Or a large salad a quarter of the size of that shown in Figure 6–2, a cup of steamed vegetables, and half of the fruit plate shown in Figure 6–2. In each case you are simply using blocks to construct the appropriate amount of insulin-promoting carbohydrate to match the amount of low-fat protein to optimize your hormonal carburetor.

If you are thinking hormonally, you know it takes fat to burn fat. So at every meal you want to add some extra fat. You must realize that fat has some very important hormonal consequences. But we want to keep the saturated fat as low as possible on a Zone Diet. That's why high-fat protein choices like the bacon don't make sense. By using low-fat protein choices, you can add monounsaturated fat of your choosing to optimize your hormonal carburetor. A great number of food items contain monounsaturated fat, as shown in Figure 6–3.

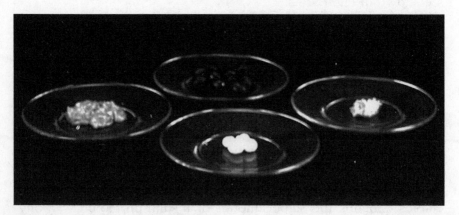

Figure 6-3. Fat Summaries

Each of these fat choices contains four blocks of primarily monounsaturated fat. Remember, fat blocks don't contain that much fat, so you are not talking about adding excessive fat to your meal. Let's start with the world's richest source of monounsaturated fat, macadamia nuts. They are essentially little balls of pure fat. That's why four macadamia nuts equal four fat blocks. Other nuts that are rich in monounsaturated fat are pistachios, cashews, and almonds. That leads us to nut butters like almond butter. Ask many gourmet chefs, and they will tell you that they always cook with almond butter instead of butter. It doesn't burn, and it presents an excellent mouth feel. And two teaspoons of almond butter are equivalent to four fat blocks. If nuts or nut butter are not your cup of tea, try olives. Twelve olives are equivalent to four fat blocks. Or 4 teaspoons of olive oil and vinegar dressing. And finally there is always avocado or my favorite, guacamole. Two tablespoons of guacamole give you four fat blocks.

Let's go back to our figures and construct balanced meals for a person who needs four blocks. It could be fourteen strips of bacon and a single Snickers bar (obviously you don't need to add any extra fat to these choices). Let's try a better choice, like 4 ounces of skinless chicken (four protein blocks), 2 ounces of pasta (four carbohydrate blocks), and four macadamia nuts (four fat blocks). Hormonally it's OK, but your carbohydrate choice isn't too high in vitamins or minerals and there's not much of it on your plate. But if you like pasta that much, then that is all you can have at that meal with that amount of protein. What if we substitute half the fruit plate in Figure 6–2 for half of the pasta? It's still four carbohydrate blocks, but now it represents a better source of vitamins. We're getting there. What if you replaced the remaining pasta with 2 cups of steamed vegetables, and in place of the four macadamia nuts, you add twelve olives to your meal for the monounsaturated fat?

A pretty hearty meal for anyone, yet less than 400 calories, assuming you eat all the vegetables. Can you see why your grandmother told you to eat all your vegetables before you leave the table? If your meal is hormonally balanced every time you eat, then you have to get enough insulin-promoting carbohydrate with each meal to balance off the protein.

What if you are a vegetarian? Simply substitute 12 ounces of firm tofu for the 4 ounces of chicken breast and do a stir fry with the vegetables, layered with twelve split olives. Then have half the fruit plate on the side as dessert. It's easy.

And, as you have seen, you get all the tough science taken care of for you when you work with blocks. All the while you are eating what you like to eat at meals; just remember to maintain the balance of blocks at every meal. Remember, too, that most people will eat a roster of about twenty items at any period in their lives. Just remember the block size of the items you like to eat and will eat. From these twenty items you can construct an infinite number of meals.

Always remind yourself that your protein requirements at a meal dictate the amount of carbohydrate before you get an insulin overload. To make it easier, use the simple one-line table in Figure 6–4.

PROTEIN COURSE	SALAD	ALCOHOL	CARBOHYDRATE MAIN COURSE	DESSERT
_____	_____	_____	_____	_____

Figure 6-4. Simplified Zone Meal Construction Template

Write down the number of protein blocks you plan to eat at your meal. Then start planning the carbohydrate content of your meal. If you want a hearty salad with that meal, then you know that will be equal to one carbohydrate block. If you want some alcohol (wine, beer, or a cocktail) with that meal, then mark down the number of drinks you plan to consume. If you want dessert with that meal, then write down the number of carbohydrate blocks it will contain. Remember that fresh fruit is still the best dessert around.

Add up all the carbohydrate blocks from these side sources of carbohydrates (salad, alcohol, or dessert) and subtract them from the protein blocks. What you have left is the number of carbohydrates remaining for your main course. Obviously if you plan to drink a lot of wine and eat a dessert, there may not be many (if any) carbohydrate blocks left for the main course. But at least you have complete control of how you want to structure a meal.

A slightly more detailed Zone meal construction template was suggested by Jill Sullivan. This template is shown in Figure 6–5 (and can also be found in Appendix D).

	PROTEIN	CARBOHYDRATE	ADDED FAT
Salad			
Protein Course			
Main Carbohydrate Course			
Dessert			
Alcohol			
Total			

Figure 6-5. Detailed Zone Meal Construction Template

For each component of the meal you plan to eat, put in the appropriate number of blocks in the various categories. When you total up all the blocks, they should in be in 1:1:1 ratio. Let's say you want to start your meal with a salad. If it is a pretty hearty dinner salad (see Appendix B for some examples), that would be one carbohydrate block. If you plan to add some salad dressing, then simply add the number of fat blocks contained in the dressing in the same category. If you plan to have some alcohol with dinner (like a glass of wine), then put the number of carbohydrate blocks you plan to consume in your total alcohol consumption in its appropriate column. If it's one glass of wine, this will be one carbohydrate block. If it's two glasses of wine, it will be two carbohydrate blocks, and so on. If you plan to have dessert (and fruit is an example of a great dessert), mark down the number of carbohydrate blocks it will contain.

Your protein course will usually consist of your protein requirement. Let's assume that you are having 6 ounces of salmon. That would be four protein blocks. Finally, what's left is to determine the size of your carbohydrate main course, which usually consists of vegetables or some grains or starches. How much salad and dessert you plan to eat plus the amount of alcohol you plan to consume, subtracted from the amount of protein, will determine the size of your carbohydrate main course.

So let's see how this hypothetical meal with 6 ounces of salmon, a glass of wine, a hearty dinner salad with a teaspoon of olive oil and vinegar dressing, and 1½ cups of steamed broccoli to go with your ¾ cup of fresh blueberries for dessert will look on your Zone meal template.

	PROTEIN	CARBOHYDRATE	ADDED FAT
Salad	0	1	1
Protein Course	4	0	0
Main Carbohydrate Course	0	1	0
Dessert	0	1	0
Alcohol	0	1	0
Total	4	4	1

From your template, you can see that the protein and carbohydrate blocks are balanced, but you are still a little short on the fat. Simply add 3 teaspoons of slivered almonds over the salmon. Now all the blocks will be in a 1:1:1 ratio and you have a perfect Zone meal.

Using this simple template, it is virtually impossible not to construct a Zone meal because it prevents you from overconsuming carbohydrates (whatever their source) relative to the amount of protein in that meal, and the template reminds you to add enough extra fat to get the best overall hormonal response for the next four to six hours.

To show you how simple this is, Table 6-1 lists a number of simple Zone meals for a person who needs four protein blocks for each meal.

Table 6-1 Typical Four-Block Zone Meals

PROTEIN	CARBOHYDRATE	ADDED FAT
6 ounces of fish	2 cups of steamed vegetables 1 piece of fruit	4 teaspoons of slivered almonds (mixed with the vegetables)
4 ounces of chicken breast	1 large salad with two tomatoes and two peppers 1 cup of steamed vegetables 1 piece of fruit	4 teaspoons of olive oil and vinegar dressing
2 soybean hamburger patties	2 cups of steamed vegetables 1 piece of fruit ¼ cup of cooked pasta	2 tablespoons of guacamole
1 cup of low-fat cottage cheese	1⅓ cups of cooked oatmeal	four macadamia nuts
Omelette consisting of 6 egg whites and 1 ounce nonfat cheese	¼ cantaloupe 1 cup strawberries 1 cup grapes	1⅓ teaspoons of olive oil (added to the omelette)

The carbohydrates in each of these five meals can be modified infinitely, either by changing the composition of the main carbohydrate course, or by reducing the amount of the main carbohydrate course by adding salads, alcoholic beverages, or dessert. Each of these basic meals can be modified with your Zone meal template. As an example, let's look at the first meal in Table 6-1, with the number of blocks in parentheses.

Table 6-2 Typical Four-Block Meal Using the Zone Meal Template

	PROTEIN	CARBOHYDRATE	ADDED FAT
Salad	-	-	-
Main Protein Course	6 ounces of fish (4)	-	-
Main Carbohydrate Course	-	2 cups of steamed vegetables (2)	4 teaspoons of slivered almonds (4)
Dessert	-	1 piece of fruit (2)	-
Alcohol	-	-	-
Total	4	4	4

Using the Food Block guides in Appendix B, making substitutions is easy. Furthermore, these five meals in Table 6-1 can be used for breakfast, lunch, or dinner. In fact, it is rare for an individual to eat more than ten different meals at home. Just take the meals you like to eat, determine their block sizes, and then readjust them with the Zone Meal template in Appendix D so that they are in the Zone.

And what about Zone snacks? Typical snacks might include the following:

- 2 ounces of low-fat cottage cheese (¼ cup or approximately 4 tablespoons), ½ piece of fruit, and three sliced olives
- 1 ounce of sliced turkey breast, 1 cup of fruit, and three almonds
- 3 ounces of firm tofu mixed with dry onion soup mix and ⅓ teaspoon of olive oil, and 2 cups of chopped raw vegetables
- 4 ounces of wine with 1 ounce of sliced cheese

That last snack sounds pretty interesting to most people. I'll let you in on a little secret: The French are actually pretty good Zone cooks (as I will explain further in Chapter 12). And the little smidgen of saturated fat in the 1 ounce of cheese is not going to kill you. I have always said, the Zone Diet is a very flexible diet. More importantly, a Zone Diet is real food!

Finally, I want to give you a couple of quick tips as you begin to construct Zone meals and snacks. Try to make all your protein choices low in fat. This will supply adequate levels of essential fatty acids to your body, while reducing your total intake of saturated fat. Make sure most of your carbohydrates come from favorable, low-glycemic and low-density carbohydrates like fruits and vegetables. Finally, when you add fat blocks, make sure they are primarily monounsaturated fat.

Don't get bogged down with attaining absolute precision when you're starting out. Simply ask yourself how you feel for the next four to six hours after a meal. If you have good mental focus and no hunger, then you were in the Zone. So instead of being obsessive about the construction of a Zone meal, pay *very* close attention to how you feel after a Zone meal. How you feel tells you whether that meal was a hormonal winner. If it was, put it into your hormonal winning cookbook that you can go back to over and over again for the same hormonal benefits, just like a drug.

But like your car, sometimes you need a tune-up or adjustment of your hormonal carburetor because not everyone is exactly the same. And here lies the power of the Zone Diet: It can be adjusted with great precision for every individual if you have the rules of how to do it. In the next chapter, I will show you how to become a master mechanic.

7

ADJUSTING YOUR HORMONAL CARBURETOR

Here's a radical thought: No two people are the same. At least this appears to be a radical thought in certain nutritional circles. The Zone Diet is based on an individual's needs, an individual's likes and tastes. More important, the Zone Diet is based on mathematics (even if it is simple math using blocks) so that it can be adjusted to a particular individual's genetics.

I say genetics because not everyone is genetically the same, especially in the insulin response to a defined intake of carbohydrates. Those genetically lucky ones (about 25 percent of the population) who have a lower insulin response to carbohydrates have a greater "slop factor." They can tolerate more carbohydrates in a meal than the average person before they move out of the Zone. On the other hand, those individuals who have a very high insulin response to carbohydrates have to watch their carbohydrate intake like a hawk.

These genetic variations to the insulin response caused by carbohydrates may be found when you look at various blood groups. For much of human evolutionary time, people were not exposed to high-density carbohydrates, such as grains. Since it takes about 10,000 to 20,000 years for even subtle genetic adaptations to take place in a population, it is not too surprising that individuals with the oldest blood groups are simply not genetically designed to handle high-density carbohydrates.

The oldest blood group is type O, which includes many native tribes such as Australian aborigines, native Hawaiians, and American

Indians. It also includes many people of Northern European ancestry. Individuals with this blood group tend to be very insulin sensitive to carbohydrates, and a high-carbohydrate diet (especially if it is rich in high-gluten grains, like wheat, used to make bread and pasta) tends to be a hormonal disaster for them.

Blood groups AB and B represent more recent genetic variations, and therefore these individuals may have a slightly diminished insulin reaction to carbohydrates. But they are not out of the woods by a long shot if they continue to consume excessive levels of carbohydrates. Finally, individuals with type A blood may represent the genetically lucky ones who can tolerate larger amounts of carbohydrates without severe overproduction of insulin. Maybe 20,000 years from now everyone will be genetically lucky, but not yet.

So how do you begin to adjust your hormonal carburetor? First by knowing when it is in tune. If you have eaten a hormonally correct meal, you won't be hungry for the next four to six hours because you will be maintaining blood sugar levels. For the same biochemical reason, you will have a very sharp mental focus. And here's the best part: You are simultaneously tapping into your stored fat as a virtually unlimited calorie source.

If your last meal put you clearly in the Zone, then mark the exact proportions of that meal in a mental diary because you can always come back to that meal in the exact same proportions again to achieve the same hormonal effect. It's a hormonal winner and one to enshrine in your personal Zone cookbook.

Great, but what happens when the carburetor is out of tune? The first warning sign is that you get hungry before the end of that four- to six-hour time period. But that symptom alone will not tell you if you have produced too much insulin or not enough insulin with your last meal, because in either case you will get hungry within two to three hours after the meal. Why is that? Well, if you are producing *too much* insulin, then blood sugar levels will be driven down, and your mental alertness drops. In other words, you get a loopy feeling. However, if your insulin levels are *too low*, then there is not enough insulin crossing the blood-brain barrier to interact with the hypothalamus to prevent the synthesis of neuropeptide Y, probably the most potent stimulator of appetite. And here is the irony. Although the brain is getting more than adequate amounts of blood sugar and thus retaining excellent mental acuity, you have a growing hunger due to the increase in neuropeptide Y levels in the brain.

So now you can play food detective to retune your carburetor. If you eat a meal and feel hungry and loopy within two to three hours (if not sooner), then that meal contained *too many* carbohydrates relative to the amount of protein. Make a mental note of the number of carbohydrate blocks you ate, and the next time you eat that same meal, maintain the same level of protein blocks, but decrease the number of carbohydrate blocks by one.

Correspondingly, if you are hungry within two to three hours, but maintain a good mental acuity, you have pushed insulin levels too low. Make a mental note of the number of carbohydrate blocks that you ate, and the next time you eat that same meal, maintain the same level of protein blocks, but increase the amount of carbohydrates blocks by one. Figure 7–1 presents these adjustment parameters in a visual format.

This very simple diagnostic chart can be used to continually fine-tune your hormonal carburetor. Regardless of how poor your last meal was, remember that you are only one meal away from getting back into the Zone by using one of your hormonally winning meals from your personal Zone cookbook.

Another way to approach this fine-tuning process is to treat it as a game. People love to play games, because they have defined rules for winning and losing and playing. The Zone Game is no different. It's a great game to play because the payoff occurs within the next four to six hours. And then it's time to play the game again. The goal of the game? Spend more time in the Zone than out of it.

Unlike most games, the Zone Game is a continuum. No matter at what involvement level you play the game, you are going to get some benefits. So to help you along, I have listed some of the basic rules to play this contest in order of increasing skill and precision. The more of the rules you follow, the better the results. Of course, to play the game well you must begin to do some hormonal thinking, and therefore take dietary responsibility in your own hands. But that's easy because on the Zone Diet you are winning along the way.

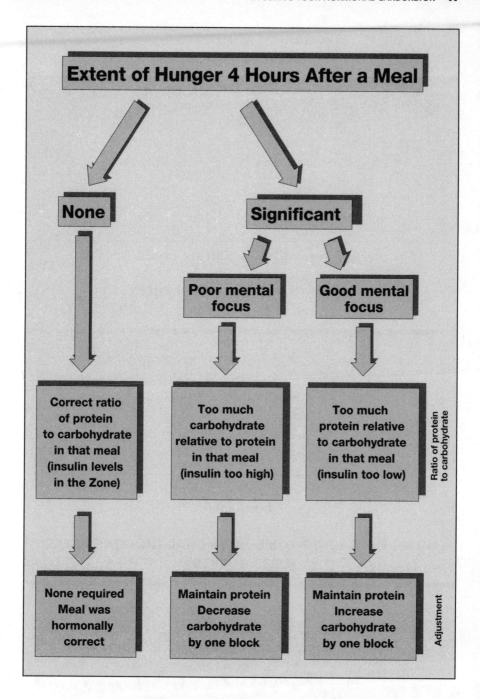

Figure 7-1. Hormonal Adjustment Diagnostic Chart

WHAT-YOUR-GRANDMOTHER-TOLD-YOU RULES
(LEVEL 1: BRONZE)

1. Drink at least 64 ounces of water per day (eight 8-ounce glasses). (Your body is composed of 70 percent water that can be easily lost.)
2. Eat more fruits and vegetables, and less pasta, breads, grains, and starches during the day.
3. Eat more frequent meals with fewer calories.
4. Eat small amounts of low-fat protein at every meal and snack.

The payoff: **You will stop gaining excess body fat.**

BEGIN-TO-PAY-ATTENTION RULES
(LEVEL 2: SILVER)

1. Determine how much protein you require per day and consume that amount.
2. Use the eyeball method to control your ratio of protein to carbohydrate at every meal.
3. Add some extra monounsaturated fat to every meal.
4. Drink 8 ounces of water thirty minutes before a meal.

The payoff: **You are going to start losing excess body fat.**

NOW-I-HAVE-TO-DO-SOME-HORMONAL-THINKING RULES
(LEVEL 3: GOLD)

1. Make sure most of your carbohydrates come from fruits and vegetables, and use grains, starches, pasta, and breads as condiments. Try to keep grains, starches, pasta, and bread to no more than 25 percent of the total carbohydrate consumed at a meal.
2. Never let more than five hours go by without eating a Zone meal or snack.
3. Always eat a Zone breakfast within one hour of rising.

4. Always have a small Zone snack before you go to bed.
5. Always have a small Zone snack thirty minutes before you exercise.

The payoff: **You're in the Zone, and you have done everything possible to achieve SuperHealth.**

Once you know how to tune up your hormonal carburetor, and decide which level of the Zone Game you want to play, then you have complete control of the quality of your life. The better the quality of life you want, the more you have to pay attention to what you eat. Although this may seem like a revelation to most people, it was pretty obvious to your grandmother.

If you put all rules into a simple graphical picture, what you get is the Zone pyramid of eating, which is shown in Figure 7–2.

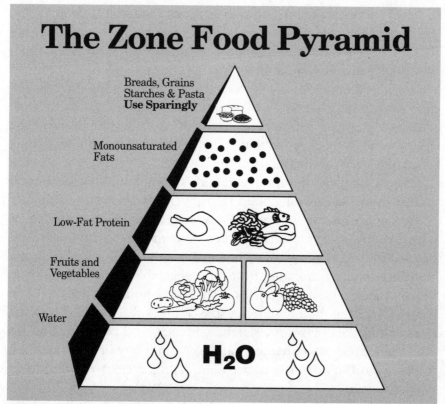

Figure 7-2. Zone Pyramid

You notice the base of the Zone pyramid is water. Your body is 70 percent water, and you need lots of it every day to maintain adequate hydration, especially on a Zone Diet in which you are burning stored body fat instead of incoming carbohydrates for energy. Water is the world's cheapest nutrient, and nobody in America drinks enough of it.

The next step of the Zone pyramid contains fruits and vegetables (the carbohydrates your grandmother told you to eat). The next rung up is low-fat protein. Notice I didn't say meat, just low-fat protein. This category includes tofu or soybean imitation meat products as well as low-fat animal sources. The next rung of the Zone pyramid is monounsaturated fat. This is hormonally neutral fat, and will have no effect on insulin. And finally at the top of the Zone pyramid to be used in moderation are grains, starches, breads, and pasta. The Zone Diet doesn't forbid these items, just asks you to treat them as condiments.

What about vitamins and minerals? As I stated in *The Zone,* the only supplement that is essential on the Zone Diet (and any diet that is low in total fat) is vitamin E. Nonetheless, there are people who feel that the food supply is compromised when it comes to vitamins and minerals. If you feel strongly about supplementation, then simply add a good multivitamin and mineral tablet at each meal. It's a cheap insurance policy. But never let the tail wag the dog. It's the Zone pyramid that is the key to SuperHealth, not some magic pill from the health food store.

Now that the Zone food pyramid is complete, let's see how it compares to the recommended U.S. government's food pyramid.

As you can clearly see, there are some major differences between the two, especially when it comes to grains, starches, pasta, and bread. Virtually every major study has found a strong association between eating fruits and vegetables and reductions in heart disease and cancer. No such correlations have ever been found for eating grains, starches, pasta, and bread. And if you still think eating lots of grains, starches, breads, and pasta is good for you, then go back to Chapter 3 and ask a mummy or read the latest research on the correlation between eating excessive amounts of pasta and cancer.

Now, if you think the rules to the Zone Game are still too hard

The Zone Food Pyramid vs. The USDA Food Pyramid

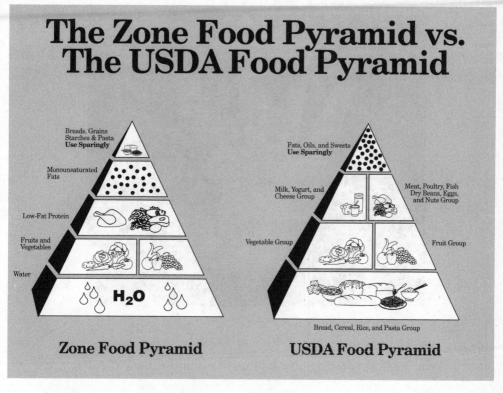

Figure 7-3. Zone Food Pyramid versus U.S. Government Food Pyramid

to remember, then simply use your hand and your eye to remind you how to play the Zone Game.

First, look at the palm of your hand and follow these simple steps:

1. Never eat any more low-fat protein than you can fit on the palm of your hand.
2. Let the volume of the low-fat protein you are going to eat determine the volume of the carbohydrates you can eat at the same time. If you're eating unfavorable carbohydrates (grains, starches, pasta, bread, etc.), then you can have the same volume portion as the low-fat protein you're eating. If you're eating favorable carbohydrates (fruits and vegetables), then you can eat double the volume of the low-fat protein portion.

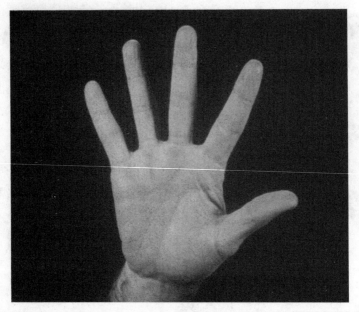

Figure 7-4. Hand Picture

Now look at the fingers on your hand and follow these simple Zone rules:

1. Eat five times a day, divided into three meals and two snacks.
2. Never let more than five hours go by without eating a Zone meal or Zone snack.
3. Try not to eat more than five blocks of any macronutrient (protein, carbohydrate, or fat) per meal.
4. Make sure that the number of carbohydrate blocks on the fingers of one hand is balanced by the number of protein blocks on the other hand at every meal or snack.

FURTHER HELPFUL HINTS

The Zone Game is simple, it's fun to play, and you get an immediate payoff if you win. It's like going to Las Vegas and playing the slot machines. Unlike Las Vegas, where you usually lose but have a good time, you try to win the Zone Game all the time and have a great time. And that's why I want to give you even more helpful tips on how to play this game.

1. Identify your personal Protein Prescription. The foundation for preparing every Zone meal and snack starts with the amount of protein that you decide to put on your plate. Be certain that when your head hits the pillow you have tried your best to consume the entire number of protein blocks that you require for the day.

2. Try having low-fat protein already prepared in your refrigerator. This can be in the form of tuna salad, sliced turkey breast, hard-boiled egg whites, low-fat cottage cheese, or a dip using firm or extra-firm tofu. It's always easy to find carbohydrates for meals or snacks, but a little advance preparation will ensure that you can always find some protein at the same time.

3. Regardless of your protein needs, never consume less than eight protein blocks per day if you're an adult.

4. Map out your daily protein requirements based on the number of protein blocks you need as determined by your Protein Prescription. Plan your Protein Prescription based on your wake-up time. Remember, *try* to eat within one hour after waking—this starts the Zone clock running. Now determine those time points throughout the day when it is necessary to refuel the body. You should never let more than five hours go by without eating, whether you're hungry or not, to maintain and sustain yourself within the Zone. In fact, the best time to eat is when you're not hungry.

5. Use the Food Block guide in Appendix B as a valuable reference tool to reduce the task of meal planning to a simple, easy-to-follow program, which allows you to create an infinite variety of Zone meals and snacks based on foods that you like to eat. Remember, you need only to match the number of protein blocks you consume at any meal or snack with the same number of carbohydrate and fat blocks to get your hormonal carburetor going.

6. Whether you have entered the Zone is ultimately not a question of percentages, totals, amounts, or the glycemic index—it's based

solely on your personal response to a meal. You don't have to be obsessive about constructing Zone meals, but pay very careful attention to how you respond to the meals you do have. Keep a mental diary of your last meal, and look for the following parameters during the next four- to six-hour cycle to determine if that meal puts you in the Zone:

- Lack of hunger.
- Lack of carbohydrate cravings.
- Good mental focus and clarity.
- Good physical energy and performance.

These are all excellent indicators that you're in the Zone. In general, two or more blocks of protein with the correct balance of carbohydrate and fat blocks should generate the desired four- to six-hour response. A one-block snack is good for two to three hours before your next meal or snack. If you're hungry after a meal, then it means you have to readjust the protein-to-carbohydrate ratio of that same meal until it generates the desired responses.

7. After the first two to three days on the Zone Diet, if you sense that you're not experiencing the benefits described earlier during any four- to six-hour interval, you're simply not in the Zone. Remember, you haven't failed, nor has the Zone Diet failed you. It's just that your particular hormonal carburetor may need some fine-tuning. But the protein-to-carbohydrate ratio is usually not to blame. It's often the amount of fat that you're *not* adding back to the diet.

    Remember, dietary fat slows the entry rate of any carbohydrate into the bloodstream. Your success entering the Zone is based on how well you control the entry rates of carbohydrates, both "favorable" and "unfavorable," for the next four- to six-hour interval. View monounsaturated fats in your diet as your ally, not your enemy. If you're having difficulty maintaining the desired four- to six-hour response, then add more monounsaturated fat to your diet at every meal and snack. A block of fat has no effect on insulin levels. Remember, it's insulin, not dietary fat, that makes you fat. This small amount of extra fat will have no effect on your rate of fat loss.

8. Do not forget the critical importance of your late-afternoon snack and especially your late-evening snack. Most people make their

mistakes by not having the late-afternoon snack, thus waiting too long before the evening meal. For example, if you had your afternoon snack at 4:30, and the evening meal is delayed until 8:30, you will begin to exit the Zone before dinner (a one-block snack is good for approximately two to three hours). You are far better off to have a one-block snack at 6:30 to keep you in the Zone until dinnertime, even if you increase the number of total protein blocks that you consume during the day. If you don't have the snack and simply hope for the best at 8:30, you may have completely exited the Zone, and will tend to consume far more carbohydrates than you need, moving you even further away from your goal.

9. Your goal is to spend as many hours of the day as you can in the Zone. Nobody is perfect. If you make a mistake (and we all have bad Zone meals, even bad Zone days), remember you're only four to six hours away from reentering the Zone. This makes the program guilt-free because you realize that you're only one Zone meal or snack away from getting back on track. This is why the late-night snack is so important. Regardless of what happened during the day, your late-night Zone snack will not only nudge you back into the Zone while you sleep, but will literally reset your biochemistry for the next morning.

10. During the first two weeks on the Zone program, try to eat only the favorable carbohydrates (fruits and vegetables). At the end of the first two weeks, reintroduce some of the unfavorable carbohydrates (grains, starches, bread, and pasta), if you desire. It doesn't mean you can't ever eat unfavorable carbohydrates, but they must be consumed in smaller amounts because they are so carbohydrate-dense. If you begin to reintroduce grains and starches and notice a decrease in performance, mental acuity, and appetite suppression, this is a pretty good indicator that you are very carbohydrate sensitive. Grains and starches should never be your primary carbohydrate source at a meal and ideally never more than 25 percent of your total carbohydrate content at a meal. It will be the balance of favorable and unfavorable carbohydrates that determines what volume of carbohydrates can be eaten with the amount of protein you plan to consume at the same meal.

11. Your primary concern is to maintain the desired four- to six-hour response regardless of the carbohydrate source. Learn to play food detective. For example, if you're not hungry before a meal, and then find yourself craving sugars and sweets two hours after a meal, you probably consumed too many carbohydrates or the wrong type of carbohydrate during your last meal.

12. Try to develop a hormonally winning cookbook. Every time you make a meal that leaves you satiated with a good mental focus for the next four to six hours, write it down. You can always come back to that meal in the exact same proportions, like a drug, to get the same hormonal effect in the future. Remember, most people will eat only twenty food items in their entire life, and eat only ten meals repetitively. Take those twenty food items you like to eat to construct an infinite number of hormonally winning Zone meals. Change the effect on your hormonal carburetor of each of your ten favorite meals into hormonal winners. For your favorite recipes like Aunt Millie's succotash, just keep tweaking the composition of that meal until you reach the Zone using the criteria in helpful hint number six. Now you have Aunt Millie's hormonally correct succotash.

13. Eat your protein portion first. Since protein stimulates glucagon, this hormone will cause the release of stored carbohydrate in the liver to keep your brain satisfied, thereby making it easy to control the carbohydrate intake. Furthermore, glucagon depresses insulin secretion, making protein your most powerful tool in controlling insulin levels.

14. Drink an 8-ounce glass of water about thirty minutes before a meal or snack. This not only decreases your hunger, but also is a good way to get the water you need on the Zone diet. Remember, on a fat-burning diet, you will need nearly 50 percent more water than you would have needed on a high-carbohydrate diet. Just as excess insulin makes your body hold on to fat, excess insulin causes water retention. As you lower insulin levels, you need to replace any water that your body is no longer retaining. This means at least eight 8-ounce glasses of water or other suitable beverages per day. Water is the cheapest nutrient on earth, yet no one drinks enough of it.

15. Chew your food thoroughly before swallowing. Does this sound like your grandmother again? Well, she was right. An intricate part of the overall digestive process begins in your mouth with the secretion of enzymes in the saliva. Remember, it's not the amount of food you eat, but the amount that is absorbed. As you age, your digestive capacity will decrease. Therefore, make every use of what you have. Furthermore, by chewing slowly, you are giving the macronutrients time to get into the bloodstream to begin generating some of those hormonal "stop eating" signals.

16. Sit down and eat, just as your grandmother always told you. You're more likely to eat less rapidly, and you might actually engage in some conversation, which allows even more time for the food to enter the bloodstream and more time for those hormonal "stop eating" signals to be sent to the brain.

17. Special Troubleshooting Hint. If all else fails, simply read *The Zone* again. Remember, *The Zone* is your dietary road map, and it takes time to learn its lessons. The principles of the Zone are not obvious. Treat it like a textbook: Mark it up, put comments in the margins, use different colored markers to highlight key passages. The more often you revisit *The Zone*, the easier it is to follow the program on a lifetime basis.

8

A WEEK IN THE ZONE

Now that you know how to spend a day in the Zone and have learned how to make adjustments to your hormonal carbure-tor, how about spending a week there? Earlier, I said that the Zone Diet is remarkably similar for both average individuals and elite, world-class athletes like Olympians. The only difference between the two populations is that the world-class athletes will require more protein (and therefore more carbohydrates) and significantly *more fat* than average individuals. As you will see, however, the strategy both these groups should use to get into the Zone is almost identical.

To show you how similar, let's compare a week of diets for (1) a typical American female who requires three blocks per meal, (2) a typical American male who requires four blocks per meal, (3) a typical female Olympian who requires five blocks per meal, and (4) a typical male Olympian who requires six blocks per meal. In addi-tion, all these people would be eating two one-block snacks, one as a late-afternoon snack and the other as a late-night snack.

The first thing that should strike you as you read these menus is that they consist of the kinds of everyday foods you already eat. The second thing is that you may find it *hard* to eat all the food. And the third thing is, paradoxically, you may be surprised to know that these meals are all low calorie. They are low calorie because they take advantage of using primarily low-density carbohydrates. As an example, a typical four-block meal contains about 400 calories.

Notice that each of these menus is broken into protein, carbo-hydrate, and fat blocks so that substitutions can by made by using the Food Block guide in Appendix B. If your own block require-ments are slightly different, make a corresponding adjustment either up or down in the proportions. For example, if you need five blocks per meal but like the four-block meal, simply increase the size of each component by about a third. On the other hand, if you need only two blocks but like a three-block meal, then decrease the size of each component in the recipe by about a third.

DAY ONE FOR THE TYPICAL AMERICAN FEMALE (THREE BLOCKS PER MEAL)

Breakfast—Scrambled Eggs

Protein:	4 egg whites or ½ cup egg substitute
	1 ounce nonfat cheese, shredded
Carbohydrate:	1 cup grapes
	½ piece rye toast
Fat:	⅔ teaspoon olive oil
	½ teaspoon fresh-ground or natural peanut butter

Cooking Instructions

Spray nonstick pan with vegetable spray. Beat eggs and shredded nonfat cheese with olive oil and add a little milk if desired. Then scramble.

Lunch—Seafood Salad Sandwich

Protein:	4½ ounces seafood (shrimp, crabmeat, or lobster)
Carbohydrate:	1 small side salad
	1 apple
	½ mini pita pocket
Fat:	1 tablespoon light mayonnaise

Note: For even better results, you can replace the mini pita pocket with a larger salad containing sliced tomatoes, green peppers, and onions (see Food Block guide), or substitute another piece of fruit. This substitution can be made for any meal that contains rye bread or a mini pita *pocket. You can also substitute 1 tablespoon olive oil and vinegar dressing for the mayonnaise.*

Cooking Instructions

Mix seafood with mayonnaise. Stuff into a mini pita pocket.

Afternoon Snack

1 ounce low-fat cheese
½ orange

Dinner—Chili

Protein:
4½ ounces lean ground meat (beef or turkey)
Sprinkling of shredded nonfat cheese

Carbohydrate:
Minced onions, chopped mushrooms, and chopped green bell pepper to taste
Chili powder, oregano, and pepper to taste
¼ cup kidney beans
1 cup tomatoes, crushed
1 peach

Fat:
1 teaspoon olive oil

Cooking Instructions

Brown meat in the olive oil with onions, mushrooms, green pepper, and spices, stirring often. Add kidney beans and tomatoes. Simmer 30 minutes or until beans are tender, stirring occasionally. Top with shredded cheese. Have the peach for dessert.

Late-Night Snack

1 ounce turkey breast, sliced
1 cup strawberries
6 peanuts

DAY TWO FOR THE TYPICAL AMERICAN FEMALE

Breakfast—Old-Fashioned Oatmeal and Bacon

Protein:	2 tablespoons protein powder (supplying 14 grams of protein)
	1 ounce Canadian bacon
Carbohydrate:	1 cup dry oatmeal plus 2 cups water
	Nutmeg and cinnamon to taste
Fat:	1 tablespoon slivered almonds

Cooking Instructions

Cook oatmeal according to package directions. After cooling, stir in protein powder and spices and top with slivered almonds. Cook Canadian bacon separately.

Lunch—Cheeseburger Lunch

Protein:	4½ ounces lean hamburger meat (less than 10 percent fat)
	1 slice reduced-fat cheese
Carbohydrate:	Tomato slice, lettuce leaf, and onion slice
	1 piece rye bread
	½ apple
Fat:	6 peanuts

Cooking Instructions

Broil hamburger to preferred degree of doneness (about 5 minutes per side for medium). Place cheese on top and broil hamburger until cheese is melted. Put cheeseburger together with the tomato, lettuce, and onion. Have the apple and peanuts for dessert.

Afternoon Snack

3 ounces firm tofu mixed with
⅓ teaspoon olive oil and
sprinkling of onion soup mix
1½ cups broccoli and green
peppers, cut for dipping

Dinner—Barbecued Chicken

Protein:
3 ounces skinless chicken
breast

Carbohydrate:
Lemon slices
Onion slices
½ teaspoon barbecue sauce
1½ cups steamed cauliflower
1 spinach salad (see Food
Block guide)
1 cup strawberries for dessert

Fat:
1 tablespoon olive oil and
vinegar dressing

Cooking Instructions

Preheat oven to 450 degrees. Cover the chicken breast with slices of lemon and onion. Bake for 15 minutes. Reduce heat to 350 degrees. Baste with barbecue sauce. Cook for 10–15 minutes or until done.

Late-Night Snack

1 ounce reduced-fat cheese
1 peach
3 olives

DAY THREE FOR THE TYPICAL AMERICAN FEMALE

Breakfast—Fruit Salad

Protein:	¾ cup low-fat cottage cheese
Carbohydrate:	1 cup strawberries
	¾ cup cantaloupe, cubed
	½ cup grapes
Fat:	3 macadamia nuts, crushed

Cooking Instructions
    Mix together and enjoy.

Lunch—Chef Salad

Protein:	1½ ounces deli-style ham
	1½ ounces deli-style turkey breast
	1 ounce reduced-fat cheese
Carbohydrate:	1 large tossed green salad (see Food Block guide)
	1 nectarine for dessert
Fat:	1 tablespoon olive oil and vinegar dressing

Afternoon Snack

¼ cup low-fat cottage cheese mixed with ½ cup diced pineapple

Dinner—Foiled Fish

Protein:	4½ ounces fish fillet of your choice (flounder is suggested)
Carbohydrate:	Freshly ground pepper to taste
	Squirt of lemon juice
	Onion to taste, chopped
	1 cup cooked asparagus
	1 tossed salad (see Food Block guide)

	1 plum for dessert
Fat:	1 tablespoon olive oil and
	vinegar dressing
	Sprinkling of Parmesan cheese

Cooking Instructions

Tear off a good-sized piece of foil. Spray the center lightly with vegetable spray. Put the fish in the center of the foil with the onion, pepper, lemon juice, and cheese. Fold foil over the fish, leaving space around the fish. Carefully turn up and seal the sides and the middle so that juices don't leak out. Bake in a 425-degree oven for 18 minutes. When done, carefully open the foil to prevent steam burns.

Late-Night Snack

1 ounce turkey breast, sliced
½ cup grapes
1 macadamia nut

DAY FOUR FOR THE TYPICAL AMERICAN FEMALE

Breakfast—Yogurt and Fruit

Protein:	1 cup plain low-fat yogurt
	1 ounce lean Canadian bacon
Carbohydrate:	1 cup strawberries
Fat:	1 tablespoon slivered almonds

Cooking Instructions

Mix fruit with yogurt and top with slivered almonds. Cook Canadian bacon separately.

Lunch—Grilled Chicken Salad

Protein:	3 ounces grilled chicken
Carbohydrate:	2 cups romaine lettuce
	¼ cup mushrooms, sliced

¼ cup tomatoes, sliced
¼ cup onions, chopped
Lemon juice to tase
Garlic powder
Dash Worcestershire sauce
Pepper to taste
Sprinkling of Parmesan cheese
1 orange

Fat: 1 tablespoon olive oil and
                                  vinegar dressing

Cooking Instructions

Prepare the salad. Drizzle salad dressing over the salad. Squeeze the lemon over the salad. Season with garlic powder and Worcestershire sauce, and grind in fresh pepper. Toss until well combined. Place grilled chicken on top and sprinkle cheese. Have the orange for dessert.

Afternoon Snack

1 ounce cheese
½ apple

Dinner—Pork Medallions and Apples

Protein: 3 ounces pork medallions or
                                 thinly sliced pork chops

Carbohydrate: ½ apple, sliced
                                   Rosemary to taste
                                   Dijon mustard to taste
                                   1 tablespoon white wine
                                   ¼ cup water
                                   1½ cups steamed broccoli
                                   1 spinach salad (see Food
                                   Block guide)

Fat: 1 tablespoon olive oil and
                                  vinegar dressing

Cooking Instructions

Put pork into baking dish in a single layer. Top with apple slices, rosemary, and mustard. Pour wine and water around the pork. Bake at 450 degrees for 15 minutes. Baste the pork with pan juices. Reduce heat to 350 degrees and continue cooking for 10–15 minutes or until pork is white, not pink, inside.

Late-Night Snack

1 ounce soft cheese
4 ounces red wine

DAY FIVE FOR THE TYPICAL AMERICAN FEMALE

Breakfast—French Toast Sticks

Protein:	4 egg whites or ½ cup egg substitute
	1 ounce extra-lean Canadian bacon
Carbohydrate:	1 slice whole grain bread
	1 cup strawberries, sliced
Fat:	1 tablespoon slivered almonds

Cooking Instructions

Cook the Canadian bacon separately. Cut bread into sticks and soak in beaten eggs. (Scramble any egg mixture that remains.) Spray a nonstick pan with vegetable spray. Over medium-low heat, cook breadsticks, turning often, until done. Top with sliced strawberries and slivered almonds.

Lunch—Chicken Salad Sandwich

Protein:	3 ounces cooked chicken breast, shredded
Carbohydrate:	Celery, chopped
	½ cup grapes
	Lettuce
	Tomato slice

	1 piece rye bread or 1 mini pita pocket
Fat:	1 tablespoon light mayonnaise

Cooking Instructions

Mix shredded chicken with mayonnaise, celery, and grapes. Put into mini pita pocket and add lettuce and tomato slice.

Afternoon Snack

½ tablespoon guacamole wrapped in 1 ounce sliced turkey

½ cup grapes

Dinner—Meatloaf

Protein:	4½ ounces lean ground beef (less than 10 percent fat) or ground turkey
	2 tablespoons egg substitute
Carbohydrate:	1 tablespoon ketchup
	¼ cup onions, chopped
	1 teaspoon bread crumbs
	Pepper to taste
	Dash Worcestershire sauce
	1½ cups cooked zucchini
	½ apple
	1 tossed salad (see Food Block guide)
Fat:	1 tablespoon olive oil and vinegar dressing

Cooking Instructions

Mix ground meat, egg substitute, ketchup, onions, bread crumbs, pepper, and Worcestershire sauce. Form into a shallow loaf and place in microwave-safe dish. Cover with waxed paper. Microwave on medium for 10–15 minutes or until done. Have the zucchini as a side dish and eat the apple for dessert.

Late-Night Snack

1 ounce turkey breast, sliced
1 cup strawberries
3 almonds

DAY SIX FOR THE TYPICAL AMERICAN FEMALE

Breakfast—Skillet Hash

Protein:	3 ounces cooked lean ham, chicken, or beef
Carbohydrate:	⅓ cup cooked potato, diced
	1 cup tomato, chopped
	Green bell pepper, onions, and mushrooms to taste, chopped
	Salt and pepper to taste
	Dash Worcestershire sauce
	¼ cantaloupe
Fat:	1 teaspoon olive oil

Cooking Instructions

In a nonstick pan, sauté green pepper, onions, and mushrooms in olive oil until tender. Add cooked meat, potato, vegetables, spices, and Worcestershire sauce. Cook, stirring, until heated through. Have cantaloupe as side dish.

Lunch—BLT Sandwich

Protein:	2 ounces cooked extra-lean Canadian bacon
	1 ounce nonfat cheese
Carbohydrate:	1 slice rye bread
	Lettuce and sliced tomato
	½ orange
Fat:	1 teaspoon light mayonnaise
	6 olives

Afternoon Snack

> 2 ounces low-fat cottage cheese
> ½ cup pineapple, diced
> 1 teaspoon slivered almonds

Dinner—Quick Turkey Dinner

Protein:	4½ ounces deli-style turkey breast or 3 ounces cooked skinless turkey breast
Carbohydrate:	1½ cups steamed broccoli
	½ cup boiled and drained onions
	½ cup cranberries
Fat:	1 tablespoon slivered almonds (sprinkled on the broccoli)

Late-Night Snack

> 1 ounce turkey breast, sliced
> 1 cup strawberries
> 3 olives

DAY SEVEN FOR THE TYPICAL AMERICAN FEMALE

Breakfast—Scrambled Eggs Benedict

Protein:	1 ounce lean Canadian bacon
	4 large egg whites or ½ cup egg substitute
Carbohydrate:	½ English muffin
	½ grapefruit
Fat:	1 teaspoon olive oil

Cooking Instructions

Beat egg whites and olive oil with a little milk if desired. Spray a nonstick pan with vegetable spray and then scramble the eggs. Toast the English muffin. Cook the Canadian bacon, place on the toasted muffin, and top with the eggs.

Lunch—Turkey in a Pocket

Protein: 4½ ounces deli-style turkey breast or 3 ounces cooked turkey breast

Carbohydrate: 1 mini pita pocket
½ green bell pepper, chopped
1 plum

Fat: 1½ tablespoons guacamole

Afternoon Snack

2 hard-boiled egg whites
½ apple
3 almonds

Dinner—Broiled Salmon

Protein: 4½ ounces salmon fillet

Carbohydrate: Rosemary to taste
Tarragon to taste
Dill to taste
Lemon (optional)
1 cup cooked zucchini
2 tomatoes, split, sprinkled with Parmesan cheese, and broiled
½ apple for dessert

Fat: 1 teaspoon olive oil

Cooking Instructions

Rub the fillet with the herbs and then brush with olive oil. Broil for 10 minutes per inch of thickness, turning and basting once. Garnish with lemon if desired. Have the apple for dessert.

Late-Night Snack

1 ounce turkey breast, sliced
1 cup strawberries
½ tablespoon guacamole

DAY ONE FOR THE TYPICAL AMERICAN MALE
(FOUR BLOCKS PER MEAL)

Breakfast—Scrambled Eggs

Protein:	6 egg whites or ¾ cup egg substitute
	1 ounce nonfat cheese, shredded
Carbohydrate:	1 cup grapes
	1 piece rye toast
Fat:	1 teaspoon olive oil
	½ teaspoon fresh-ground or natural peanut butter

Cooking Instructions

Spray a nonstick pan with vegetable spray. Beat the eggs and shredded nonfat cheese with the olive oil and add a little milk if desired. Then scramble. Spread peanut butter on the toast.

Lunch—Seafood Salad Sandwich

Protein:	6 ounces seafood (shrimp, crabmeat, or lobster)
Carbohydrate:	1 small side salad
	1 apple
	1 piece whole rye bread or 1 mini pita pocket
Fat:	1 tablespoon light mayonnaise
	3 olives, chopped

Note: For even better results, you can replace the rye bread or mini pita pocket with a larger salad containing sliced tomatoes, green bell peppers, and onions (see Food Block guide), or substitute another piece of fruit. This substitution can be made for any meal that contains rye bread or a mini pita pocket. You can also substitute 1 tablespoon olive oil and vinegar dressing for the mayonnaise.

Cooking Instructions

Mix seafood with mayonnaise. Stuff into a mini pita pocket.

Afternoon Snack

1 ounce turkey breast
½ orange
3 almonds

Dinner—Chili

Protein:
6 ounces lean ground meat
(beef or turkey)
Sprinkling of shredded nonfat
cheese

Carbohydrate:
Minced onions, chopped
mushrooms, and chopped
green bell pepper to taste
Chili powder, oregano, and
pepper to taste
½ cup kidney beans
1 cup tomatoes, crushed
1 peach

Fat:
1⅓ teaspoons olive oil

Cooking Instructions

Brown the meat in the olive oil with onions, mushrooms, green pepper, and spices, stirring often. Add kidney beans and tomatoes. Simmer 30 minutes or until the beans are tender, stirring occasionally. Top with shredded cheese. Have the peach for dessert.

Late-Night Snack

1 ounce turkey breast, sliced
1 cup strawberries
6 peanuts

DAY TWO FOR THE TYPICAL AMERICAN MALE

Breakfast—Old-Fashioned Oatmeal and Bacon

Protein:	3 tablespoons protein powder (supplying 21 grams of protein)
	1 ounce Canadian bacon
Carbohydrate:	1 cup dry oatmeal plus 2 cups water
	¼ cup unsweetened applesauce
	Nutmeg and cinnamon to taste
Fat:	4 teaspoons slivered almonds

Cooking Instructions

Cook oatmeal according to package directions. After cooling, stir in protein powder, applesauce, and spices, and top with slivered almonds. Cook the Canadian bacon separately.

Lunch—Cheeseburger Lunch

Protein:	6 ounces lean hamburger meat (less than 10 percent fat)
	1 slice reduced-fat cheese
Carbohydrate:	Tomato slice, lettuce leaf, and onion slice
	1 piece rye bread
	1 apple
Fat:	4 macadamia nuts

Cooking Instructions

Broil hamburger to preferred degree of doneness (about 5 minutes per side for medium). Place cheese on top and broil hamburger until cheese is melted. Put cheeseburger together with the tomato, lettuce, and onion. Have the apple and nuts for dessert.

Afternoon Snack

3 ounces firm tofu mixed with
⅓ teaspoon olive oil and
sprinkling of onion soup mix
1½ cups broccoli and green
peppers, chopped

Dinner—Barbecued Chicken

Protein: 4 ounces skinless chicken
breast
Carbohydrate: Lemon slices
Onion slices
½ teaspoon barbecue sauce
1½ cups steamed cauliflower
1½ cups steamed zucchini
1 tossed salad (see Food Block
guide)
1 cup strawberries for dessert
Fat: 4 teaspoons olive oil and
vinegar dressing

Cooking Instructions

Preheat oven to 450 degrees. Cover the chicken breast with slices of lemon and onion. Bake for 15 minutes. Reduce heat to 350 degrees. Baste with barbecue sauce. Cook for 10–15 minutes or until done.

Late-Night Snack

1 ounce nonfat cheese
1 peach
3 olives

DAY THREE FOR THE TYPICAL AMERICAN MALE

Breakfast—Fruit Salad

Protein:	1 cup low-fat cottage cheese
Carbohydrate:	1 cup strawberries
	¾ cup cantaloupe, cubed
	1 cup grapes
Fat:	4 macadamia nuts, crushed

Cooking Instructions
Mix together and enjoy.

Lunch—Chef Salad

Protein:	1½ ounces deli-style ham
	3 ounces deli-style turkey breast
	1 ounce reduced-fat cheese
Carbohydrate:	1 large tossed green salad (see Food Block guide)
	1 nectarine and 1 plum for dessert
Fat:	4 teaspoons olive oil and vinegar dressing

Afternoon Snack

¼ cup low-fat cottage cheese
½ cup pineapple, diced
1 teaspoon slivered almonds

Dinner—Foiled Fish

Protein:	6 ounces fish fillet of your choice (flounder is suggested)
Carbohydrate:	Freshly ground pepper to taste
	Squirt of lemon juice

	Onion to taste, chopped
	2 cups cooked asparagus
	1 tossed salad
	1 cup strawberries, sliced, for dessert
Fat:	Sprinkling of Parmesan cheese
	4 teaspoons olive oil and vinegar dressing

Cooking Instructions

Tear off a good-sized piece of foil. Spray the center lightly with vegetable spray. Put the fish in the center of the foil with the onion, pepper, lemon juice, and cheese. Fold foil over the fish, leaving space around the fish. Carefully turn up and seal the sides and the middle so that juices don't leak out. Bake in a 425-degree oven for 18 minutes. When done, carefully open the foil to prevent steam burns.

Late-Night Snack

1 ounce turkey breast, sliced
½ cup grapes
1 macadamia nut

DAY FOUR FOR THE TYPICAL AMERICAN MALE

Breakfast—Yogurt and Fruit

Protein:	1½ cups plain low-fat yogurt
	1 ounce lean Canadian bacon
Carbohydrate:	1 cup strawberries, sliced
Fat:	4 teaspoons slivered almonds

Cooking Instructions

Mix fruit with yogurt and top with slivered almonds. Cook the Canadian bacon separately.

Lunch—Grilled Chicken Salad

Protein:	4 ounces grilled chicken
Carbohydrate:	3 cups romaine lettuce
	½ cup mushrooms, sliced
	½ cup tomatoes, sliced
	½ cup onions, chopped
	Lemon juice to taste
	Sprinkling of garlic powder
	Dash Worcestershire sauce
	Pepper to taste
	Sprinkling of Parmesan cheese
	1 breadstick
	1 apple
Fat:	4 teaspoons olive oil and vinegar dressing

Cooking Instructions

Prepare the salad. Drizzle salad dressing over the salad. Squeeze the lemon over the salad. Season with garlic powder and Worcestershire sauce, and grind in fresh pepper. Toss until well combined. Place grilled chicken on top and sprinkle with cheese and crumbled breadstick. Have the apple for dessert.

Afternoon Snack

1 ounce nonfat cheese
½ apple
6 peanuts

Dinner—Pork Medallions and Apples

Protein:	4 ounces pork medallions or thinly sliced pork chops
Carbohydrate:	1 apple, sliced
	Rosemary to taste
	Dijon mustard to taste
	1 tablespoon white wine
	¼ cup water

1½ cups steamed broccoli

1 spinach salad (see Food
Block guide)

Fat: 4 teaspoons olive oil and
vinegar dressing

Cooking Instructions

Put pork into baking dish in a single layer. Top with apple slices, rosemary, and mustard. Pour wine and water around the pork. Bake at 450 degrees for 15 minutes. Baste the pork with pan juices. Reduce heat to 350 degrees and continue cooking for 10–15 minutes or until pork is white, not pink, inside.

Late-Night Snack

1 ounce soft cheese
4 ounces red wine

DAY FIVE FOR THE TYPICAL AMERICAN MALE

Breakfast—French Toast Sticks

Protein: 6 egg whites or ¾ cup egg
substitute

1 ounce extra-lean Canadian
bacon

Carbohydrate: 1 slice whole grain bread

1 cup strawberries, sliced

¼ cantaloupe, cubed

Fat: 4 teaspoons slivered almonds

Cooking Instructions

Cook the Canadian bacon separately. Cut bread into sticks and soak in beaten eggs. (Scramble any egg mixture that remains.) Spray a nonstick pan with vegetable spray. Over medium-low heat, cook breadsticks, turning often until done. Top with sliced strawberries and slivered almonds. Have the cantaloupe as a side dish.

Lunch—Chicken Salad Sandwich

Protein:	4 ounces cooked chicken breast, shredded
Carbohydrate:	Celery, chopped
	1 cup grapes
	Lettuce
	Tomato slice
	1 piece rye bread or 1 mini pita pocket
Fat:	4 teaspoons light mayonnaise

Cooking Instructions

Mix shredded chicken with mayonnaise, celery, and grapes. Put into mini pita pocket and add lettuce and tomato slice.

Afternoon Snack

1 tablespoon guacamole wrapped in 1 ounce sliced turkey
½ cup grapes

Dinner—Meatloaf

Protein:	3 ounces lean ground beef (less than 10 percent fat)
	3 ounces ground turkey
	2 tablespoons egg substitute
Carbohydrate:	1 tablespoon ketchup
	½ cup onions, chopped
	1 teaspoon bread crumbs
	Pepper to taste
	Dash Worcestershire sauce
	1½ cups cooked zucchini
	1 apple
	1 tossed salad
Fat:	4 teaspoons olive oil and vinegar dressing

Cooking Instructions

Mix ground meat, egg substitute, ketchup, onions, bread crumbs, pepper, and Worcestershire sauce. Form into a shallow loaf and place in microwave-safe dish. Cover with waxed paper. Microwave on medium for 10–15 minutes or until done. Have the zucchini as a side dish and eat the apple for dessert.

Late-Night Snack

> 1 ounce turkey breast, sliced
> 1 cup strawberries
> 6 peanuts

DAY SIX FOR THE TYPICAL AMERICAN MALE

Breakfast—Skillet Hash

Protein:	4 ounces cooked lean ham, chicken, or beef
Carbohydrate:	⅓ cup cooked potato, diced
	1 cup tomato, chopped
	Green bell pepper, onions, and mushrooms to taste, chopped
	Salt and pepper to taste
	Dash Worcestershire sauce
	½ cantaloupe
Fat:	1⅓ teaspoons olive oil

Cooking Instructions

In a nonstick pan, sauté green pepper, onions, and mushrooms in olive oil until tender. Add cooked meat, potato, tomato, spices, and Worcestershire sauce. Cook, stirring, until heated through. Have cantaloupe as side dish.

Lunch—BLT Sandwich

Protein:	3 ounces cooked extra-lean Canadian bacon
	1 ounce nonfat cheese

Carbohydrate:
1 slice rye bread
Lettuce and sliced tomato
1 orange

Fat:
1 teaspoon light mayonnaise
3 macadamia nuts

Afternoon Snack

2 ounces low-fat cottage cheese
½ cup pineapple, diced
3 olives, chopped

Dinner—Quick Turkey Dinner

Protein:
6 ounces deli-style turkey
    breast or 4 ounces cooked
    skinless turkey breast

Carbohydrate:
1½ cups steamed broccoli
1 cup boiled and drained
    onions
½ cup cranberries

Fat:
4 teaspoons slivered almonds

Late-Night Snack

1 ounce turkey breast, sliced
1 cup strawberries
6 peanuts

DAY SEVEN FOR THE TYPICAL AMERICAN MALE

Breakfast—Scrambled Eggs Benedict

Protein:
2 ounces lean Canadian bacon
4 large egg whites or ½ cup
    egg substitute

Carbohydrate:
½ English muffin
1 orange

Fat:
1⅓ teaspoons olive oil

Cooking Instructions

Beat egg whites and olive oil with a little milk if desired. Spray a nonstick pan with vegetable spray and then scramble the eggs. Toast the English muffin. Cook the Canadian bacon, place on the toasted muffin, and then top with the eggs.

Lunch—Turkey in a Pocket

Protein:	6 ounces deli-style turkey breast or 4 ounces cooked turkey breast
Carbohydrate:	1 mini pita pocket
	1 green bell pepper, chopped
	1 tomato, sliced
	1 plum
Fat:	2 tablespoons guacamole

Afternoon Snack

2 hard-boiled egg whites
½ apple
1 celery stick stuffed with ½ teaspoon fresh-ground or natural peanut butter

Dinner—Broiled Salmon

Protein:	6 ounces salmon fillet
Carbohydrate:	Rosemary to taste
	Tarragon to taste
	Dill to taste
	Lemon (optional)
	1½ cups cooked zucchini
	2 tomatoes, split and sprinkled with Parmesan cheese
	1 apple for dessert
Fat:	1⅓ teaspoons olive oil

Cooking Instructions

Rub the fillet with the herbs, and then brush with olive oil. Broil for 10 minutes per inch of thickness, turning and basting once. Garnish with lemon if desired. Have the apple for dessert.

Late-Night Snack

1 ounce turkey breast, sliced
1 cup strawberries
1 teaspoon slivered almonds

DAY ONE FOR THE TYPICAL AMERICAN FEMALE OLYMPIC ATHLETE (FIVE BLOCKS PER MEAL)

Breakfast—Scrambled Eggs

Protein:	6 egg whites or ¾ cup egg substitute
	2 ounces nonfat cheese, shredded
Carbohydrate:	1½ cups grapes
	1 piece rye toast
Fat:	2 teaspoons olive oil
	2 teaspoons fresh-ground or natural peanut butter

Cooking Instructions

Spray a nonstick pan with vegetable spray. Beat the eggs and shredded nonfat cheese with the olive oil and add a little milk if desired. Then scramble. Spread peanut butter on the toast.

Lunch—Seafood Salad Sandwich

Protein:	7½ ounces seafood (shrimp, crabmeat, or lobster)
Carbohydrate:	1 small side salad
	½ apple
	1 orange

	1 piece whole rye bread or mini pita pocket
Fat:	5 teaspoons light mayonnaise
	5 macadamia nuts

Note: For even better results, you can replace the rye bread or mini pita pocket with a larger salad containing sliced tomatoes, green peppers, and onions (see Food Block guide), or substitute another piece of fruit. This substitution can be made for any meal that contains rye bread or a mini pita pocket. You can also substitute 5 teaspoons olive oil and vinegar dressing for the mayonnaise and serve the seafood on top of the salad.

Cooking Instructions

Mix seafood with mayonnaise. Stuff into a mini pita pocket.

Afternoon Snack

1 ounce low-fat cheese
½ orange
12 peanuts

Dinner—Chili

Protein:	6 ounces lean ground meat (beef or turkey)
	1 ounce nonfat cheese, shredded
Carbohydrate:	Minced onions, chopped mushrooms, and chopped green bell pepper to taste
	Chili powder, oregano, and pepper to taste
	½ cup kidney beans
	1 cup tomatoes, crushed
	1 nectarine
Fat:	3 teaspoons olive oil
	3 olives

Cooking Instructions

Brown the meat in the olive oil with onions, mushrooms, green pepper, olives, and spices, stirring often. Add kidney beans and tomatoes. Simmer 30 minutes or until beans are tender, stirring occasionally. Top with shredded cheese. Have the nectarine for dessert.

Late-Night Snack

> 1 ounce turkey breast, sliced
> 1 cup strawberries
> 1 tablespoon guacamole

DAY TWO FOR THE TYPICAL AMERICAN FEMALE OLYMPIC ATHLETE

Breakfast–Old-Fashioned Oatmeal and Bacon

Protein:	4 tablespoons protein powder (providing 21 grams of protein)
	2 ounces Canadian bacon
Carbohydrate:	1⅓ cups dry oatmeal plus 2½ cups water
	Nutmeg and cinnamon to taste
	¼ cantaloupe
Fat:	2 tablespoons slivered almonds
	1⅓ teaspoons olive oil

Cooking Instructions

Cook oatmeal according to package directions. After cooling, stir in protein powder, spices, and olive oil and top with slivered almonds. Cook the Canadian bacon separately. Have the cantaloupe as a side dish.

Lunch—Cheeseburger Lunch

Protein:	7½ ounces lean hamburger meat (less than 10 percent fat)
	1 slice reduced-fat cheese
Carbohydrate:	Tomato slice, lettuce leaf, and onion slice
	1 piece rye bread
	1 pear
	1 kiwi
Fat:	1 teaspoon reduced-fat mayonnaise
	9 macadamia nuts

Cooking Instructions

Broil the hamburger to preferred degree of doneness (about 5 minutes per side for medium). Put cheese on hamburger and broil until melted. Have the pear, kiwi, and macadamia nuts for dessert.

Afternoon Snack

3 ounces firm tofu mixed with
⅔ teaspoon olive oil and
sprinkling of onion soup mix
2 cups broccoli and green
peppers, chopped

Dinner—Barbecued Chicken

Protein:	5 ounces skinless chicken breast
Carbohydrate:	Lemon slices
	Onion slices
	1 teaspoon barbecue sauce
	1½ cups steamed cauliflower
	¼ cup cooked rice
	1 tossed salad (see Food Block guide)
	2 cups strawberries for dessert

Fat: 3 tablespoons olive oil and
                                    vinegar dressing
                                  6 peanuts, crushed

Cooking Instructions
Preheat oven to 450 degrees. Cover chicken breast with slices of lemon and onion. Bake for 15 minutes. Reduce heat to 350 degrees. Baste with barbecue sauce. Cook for 10–15 minutes or until done. Sprinkle peanuts on top of the salad.

Late-Night Snack

1 ounce reduced-fat cheese
1 peach
6 olives

DAY THREE FOR THE TYPICAL AMERICAN FEMALE OLYMPIC ATHLETE

Breakfast—Fruit Salad

Protein: 1¼ cups low-fat cottage cheese
Carbohydrate: 2 cups strawberries
                  ¾ cup cantaloupe, cubed
                  1 cup grapes
Fat: 10 macadamia nuts, crushed

Cooking Instructions
Mix together and enjoy.

Lunch—Chef Salad

Protein: 3 ounces deli-style ham
                  3 ounces deli-style turkey
                    breast
                  1 ounce reduced-fat cheese
Carbohydrate: 1 large tossed green salad

2 nectarines for dessert

Fat: 3 tablespoons olive oil and
vinegar dressing
1 teaspoon slivered
almonds

Afternoon Snack

2 ounces low-fat cottage cheese
½ cup pineapple, diced
2 teaspoons slivered almonds

Dinner—Foiled Fish

Protein: 7½ ounces fish fillet of your
choice (flounder is suggested)

Carbohydrate: Freshly ground pepper to taste
Squirt of lemon juice
1 onion, chopped
2 cups cooked asparagus
¼ cup cooked pasta
1 tossed salad

Fat: 3 tablespoons olive oil and
vinegar dressing
Sprinkling of Parmesan cheese
3 almonds

Cooking Instructions

Tear off a good-sized piece of foil. Spray the center lightly with vegetable spray. Put the fish in the center of the foil with the onion, pepper, lemon juice, and cheese. Fold foil over the fish, leaving space around the fish. Carefully turn up and seal the sides and the middle so that juices don't leak out. Bake in a 425-degree oven for 18 minutes. When done, carefully open the foil to prevent steam burns.

Late-Night Snack

1 ounce turkey breast, sliced
½ cup grapes
2 macadamia nuts

DAY FOUR FOR THE TYPICAL AMERICAN FEMALE OLYMPIC ATHLETE

Breakfast—Yogurt and Fruit

Protein:	Roughly ⅓ ounce protein powder (providing 7 grams of protein)
	1½ cups plain low-fat yogurt
	2 ounces lean Canadian bacon or 6 turkey bacon strips
Carbohydrate:	¾ cup cantaloupe, cubed
	½ cup blueberries
Fat:	5 teaspoons slivered almonds
	5 macadamia nuts, crushed

Cooking Instructions

Mix fruit and protein powder with yogurt and top with slivered almonds and crushed macadamia nuts. Cook the Canadian bacon separately.

Lunch—Grilled Chicken Salad

Protein:	5 ounces grilled chicken
Carbohydrate:	3 cups romaine lettuce
	½ cup mushrooms, sliced
	¾ cup tomatoes, sliced
	½ cup onions, chopped
	Lemon juice to taste
	Sprinkling of garlic powder
	Dash Worcestershire sauce
	Pepper to taste
	1 apple
	½ cup grapes
	1 breadstick
Fat:	3 tablespoons olive oil and vinegar dressing
	1 teaspoon slivered almonds
	Sprinkling of Parmesan cheese

Cooking Instructions

Prepare the salad. Drizzle salad dressing over the salad. Squeeze the lemon over the salad. Season with garlic powder and Worcestershire sauce, and grind in fresh pepper. Toss until well combined. Place grilled chicken on top, and sprinkle with slivered almonds and Parmesan cheese.

Afternoon Snack

> 1 ounce nonfat cheese
> ½ apple
> 12 peanuts

Dinner—Pork Medallions and Apples

Protein: 5 ounces pork medallions or
                       thinly sliced pork chops

Carbohydrate: 1 apple, sliced
                    Rosemary to taste
                    Dijon mustard to taste
                    1 tablespoon white wine
                    ¼ cup water
                    1½ cups steamed broccoli
                    1 spinach salad (see Food
                       Block guide)
                    ½ orange as dessert

Fat: 3 tablespoons olive oil and
                       vinegar dressing
                    6 peanuts

Cooking Instructions

Put pork into baking dish in a single layer. Top with apple slices, rosemary, and mustard. Pour wine and water around the pork. Bake at 450 degrees for 15 minutes. Baste the pork with pan juices. Reduce heat to 350 degrees and continue cooking for 10–15 minutes or until pork is white, not pink, inside.

Late-Night Snack

> 1 ounce soft cheese
> 4 ounces red wine

DAY FIVE FOR THE TYPICAL AMERICAN FEMALE OLYMPIC ATHLETE

Breakfast—French Toast Sticks

Protein:	6 egg whites or ¾ cup egg substitute
	2 ounces extra-lean Canadian bacon
Carbohydrate:	1½ slices whole grain bread
	2 cups strawberries, sliced
Fat:	2 tablespoons slivered almonds
	1⅓ teaspoons olive oil

Cooking Instructions

Cut bread into sticks and soak in beaten eggs. (Scramble any egg mixture that remains.) Spray a nonstick pan with vegetable spray. Over medium-low heat, cook breadsticks, turning often, until done. Top with sliced strawberries and slivered almonds. Sauté Canadian bacon in olive oil.

Lunch—Chicken Salad Sandwich

Protein:	5 ounces cooked chicken breast, shredded
Carbohydrate:	Celery, chopped
	1 cup grapes
	Lettuce
	Tomato slice
	1 piece rye bread or 1 mini pita pocket
	1 plum
Fat:	3 tablespoons light mayonnaise
	3 almonds

Cooking Instructions

Mix shredded chicken with mayonnaise, celery, and grapes. Put into mini pita pocket and add lettuce and tomato slice.

Afternoon Snack

1 tablespoon guacamole
    wrapped in 1 ounce sliced
    turkey
½ cup grapes

Dinner—Meatloaf

Protein: 7½ ounces lean ground beef
                            (less than 10 percent fat) or
                            ground turkey
                        2 tablespoons egg substitute
Carbohydrate: 1 tablespoon ketchup
                        ¼ cup onions, chopped
                        1 teaspoon bread crumbs
                        Pepper to taste
                        Dash Worcestershire sauce
                        2 cups green beans
                        1 apple as dessert
                        1 tossed salad (see Food Block
                            guide)
Fat: 3 tablespoons olive oil and
                            vinegar dressing
                        3 olives, chopped

Cooking Instructions

Mix ground meat, egg substitute, ketchup, onions, bread crumbs, pepper, and Worcestershire sauce. Form into a shallow loaf and place in microwave-safe dish. Cover with waxed paper. Microwave on medium for 15 minutes or until done. Steam green beans as a side dish. Have the apple for dessert.

Late-Night Snack

1 ounce turkey breast, sliced
1 cup strawberries
2 macadamia nuts

DAY SIX FOR THE TYPICAL AMERICAN FEMALE OLYMPIC ATHLETE

Breakfast—Skillet Hash

Protein:	5 ounces cooked lean ham
Carbohydrate:	⅓ cup cooked potato, diced
	2 cups tomato, chopped
	Green bell pepper, onions, and mushrooms to taste, chopped
	Salt and pepper to taste
	Dash Worcestershire sauce
	½ cantaloupe
Fat:	3 teaspoons olive oil
	6 peanuts

Cooking Instructions

In a nonstick pan, sauté green pepper, onions, and mushrooms in olive oil until tender. Add cooked meat, potato, tomato, spices, and Worcestershire sauce. Cook, stirring, until heated through. Have cantaloupe as side dish.

Lunch—BLT Sandwich

Protein:	3 ounces cooked extra-lean Canadian bacon
	2 ounces nonfat cheese
Carbohydrate:	2 slices rye bread
	Lettuce and sliced tomato
	½ orange
Fat:	1 teaspoon light mayonnaise
	9 macadamia nuts

Afternoon Snack

	1 ounce low-fat cottage cheese
	½ cup pineapple, diced
	12 peanuts

Dinner-Quick Turkey Dinner

Protein: 7½ ounces deli-style turkey
                            breast or 5 ounces cooked
                            skinless turkey breast

Carbohydrate: 3 cups steamed broccoli
                            1 cup boiled and drained
                            onions
                            ¼ cup cooked cranberries

Fat: 5 teaspoons slivered almonds

Cooking Instructions
Cook, and then sprinkle the slivered almonds on the broccoli.

Late-Night Snack

1 ounce turkey breast, sliced
1 cup strawberries
6 olives

DAY SEVEN FOR THE TYPICAL AMERICAN FEMALE OLYMPIC ATHLETE

Breakfast--Scrambled Eggs Benedict

Protein: 2 ounces lean Canadian bacon
                            6 large egg whites or ¾ cup
                            egg substitute

Carbohydrate: 1 English muffin
                            ½ grapefruit

Fat: 2 tablespoons olive oil
                            3 almonds

Cooking Instructions
Beat egg whites and olive oil with a little milk if desired. Spray nonstick pan with vegetable spray and then scramble the eggs. Toast the English muffin. Cook the Canadian bacon, place on the toasted muffin, and top with the eggs.

Lunch—Turkey in a Pocket

Protein:	7½ ounces deli-style turkey breast or 5 ounces cooked turkey breast
Carbohydrate:	1 mini pita pocket
	1 green bell pepper, chopped
	1 tomato, sliced
	1 cup strawberries
	1 orange
Fat:	5 tablespoons guacamole

Afternoon Snack

2 hard-boiled egg whites
½ apple
6 almonds

Dinner—Broiled Salmon

Protein:	7½ ounces salmon fillet
Carbohyrate:	Rosemary to taste
	Tarragon to taste
	Dill to taste
	Lemon (optional)
	3 cups cooked zucchini
	2 tomatoes, split, sprinkled with Parmesan cheese, and broiled
	1 apple for dessert
Fat:	2 teaspoons olive oil
	4 macadamia nuts

Cooking Instructions

Rub the fillet with the herbs, and then brush with olive oil. Broil for 10 minutes per inch of thickness, turning off and basting once. Garnish with lemon if desired. Have the apple for dessert.

Late-Night Snack

1 ounce turkey breast, sliced
1 cup strawberries
6 olives

DAY ONE FOR THE TYPICAL AMERICAN MALE OLYMPIC ATHLETE (SIX BLOCKS PER MEAL)

Breakfast—Scrambled Eggs

Protein:	8 egg whites or 1 cup egg substitute
	1 ounce nonfat cheese, shredded
	1 ounce lean Canadian bacon
Carbohydrate:	1 cantaloupe
	1 piece rye toast
Fat:	1½ teaspoons fresh-ground or natural peanut butter
	3 tablespoons olive oil

Cooking Instructions

Spray a nonstick pan with vegetable spray. Beat the eggs and shredded nonfat cheese with the olive oil and add a little milk if desired. Then scramble. Spread peanut butter on the toast.

Lunch—Seafood Salad Sandwich

Protein:	9 ounces seafood (shrimp, crabmeat, or lobster)
Carbohydrate:	1 small side salad
	1 orange
	2 pieces whole rye bread or ½ regular-sized pita pocket
Fat:	2 tablespoons light mayonnaise
	2 tablespoons olive oil and vinegar dressing

Note: For even better results, you can replace half of the rye bread or pita pocket with a larger salad containing sliced tomatoes, green pep-

pers, and onions (see Food Block guide), or substitute another piece of fruit. This substitution can be made for any meal that contains rye bread or a mini pita pocket.

Cooking Instructions

Mix seafood with mayonnaise. Stuff into a pita pocket.

Afternoon Snack

> 1 ounce low-fat cheese
> ½ orange
> 2 macadamia nuts

Dinner—Chili

Protein:	7½ ounces lean ground meat (beef or turkey)
	1 ounce nonfat cheese, shredded
Carbohydrate:	Minced onions, chopped mushrooms, and chopped green bell pepper to taste
	Chili powder, oregano, and pepper to taste
	¾ cup kidney beans
	1 cup tomatoes, crushed
	2 peaches
Fat:	4 teaspoons olive oil

Cooking Instructions

Brown the meat in olive oil with onions, mushrooms, green pepper, and spices, stirring often. Add kidney beans and tomatoes. Simmer 30 minutes or until beans are tender, stirring occasionally. Top with shredded cheese. Have the peaches for dessert.

Late-Night Snack

> 1 ounce turkey breast, sliced
> 1 cup strawberries
> 6 olives

DAY TWO FOR THE TYPICAL AMERICAN MALE OLYMPIC ATHLETE

Breakfast—Old-Fashioned Oatmeal and Bacon

Protein:	3 tablespoons protein powder (providing 21 grams of protein)
	3 ounces Canadian bacon
Carbohydrate:	1⅓ cups dry oatmeal plus 2½ cups water
	Nutmeg and cinnamon to taste
	½ cantaloupe
Fat:	4 tablespoons slivered almonds

Cooking Instructions

Cook oatmeal according to package directions. After cooling, stir in protein powder and spices, and top with slivered almonds. Cook the Canadian bacon separately.

Lunch—Cheeseburger Lunch

Protein:	7½ ounces lean hamburger meat (less than 10 percent fat)
	1 ounce reduced-fat cheese
Carbohydrate:	Tomato slice, lettuce leaf, and onion slice
	2 pieces rye bread
	1 apple
Fat:	12 macadamia nuts

Cooking Instructions

Broil hamburger to preferred degree of doneness (about 5 minutes per side for medium). Put cheese on hamburger and broil until melted. Have the apple and macadamia nuts for dessert.

Afternoon Snack

> 3 ounces firm tofu
> ⅔ teaspoon olive oil
> Sprinkling of onion soup mix
> 1½ cups broccoli and green bell pepper, chopped

Dinner—Barbecued Chicken

Protein:	6 ounces skinless chicken breast
Carbohydrate:	Lemon slices
	Onion slices
	1 teaspoon barbecue sauce
	3 cups steamed cauliflower
	1 apple
	1 cup strawberries for dessert
	1 tossed salad (see Food Block guide)
Fat:	4 tablespoons olive oil and vinegar dressing

Cooking Instructions

Preheat oven to 450 degrees. Cover the chicken breast with slices of lemon and onion. Bake for 15 minutes. Reduce heat to 350 degrees. Baste with barbecue sauce. Cook for 10–15 minutes or until done.

Late-Night Snack

> 1 ounce reduced-fat cheese
> 1 peach
> 6 olives

DAY THREE FOR THE TYPICAL AMERICAN MALE OLYMPIC ATHLETE

Breakfast—Fruit Salad

Protein:	1½ cups low-fat cottage cheese
Carbohydrate:	1 cup strawberries
	1 cup honeydew melon, cubed
	1 cup mandarin oranges
Fat:	12 macadamia nuts, crushed

Cooking Instructions
   Mix together and enjoy.

Lunch—Chef Salad

Protein:	3 ounces deli-style ham
	3 ounces deli-style turkey breast
	2 ounces reduced-fat cheese
Carbohydrate:	1 large tossed green salad (see Food Block guide)
	2 nectarines and 1 plum for dessert
Fat:	4 tablespoons olive oil and vinegar dressing

Afternoon Snack

2 ounces low-fat cottage cheese
½ cup pineapple, diced
6 almonds

Dinner—Foiled Fish

Protein:	9 ounces fish fillet of your choice (flounder is suggested)
Carbohydrate:	Freshly ground pepper to taste
	Squirt of lemon juice

	Onion to taste, chopped
	2 cups cooked asparagus
	½ cup cooked pasta
	1 spinach salad (see Food Block guide)
	1 tangerine
Fat:	Sprinkling of Parmesan cheese
	4 tablespoons olive oil and vinegar dressing

Cooking Instructions

Tear off a good-sized piece of foil. Spray the center lightly with vegetable spray. Put the fish in the center of the foil with the onion, pepper, lemon juice, and cheese. Fold foil over the fish, leaving space around the fish. Carefully turn up and seal the sides and the middle so that juices don't leak out. Bake in a 425-degree oven for 18 minutes. When done, carefully open the foil to prevent steam burns.

Late-Night Snack

1 ounce turkey breast, sliced
½ cup grapes
2 macadamia nuts

DAY FOUR FOR THE TYPICAL AMERICAN MALE OLYMPIC ATHLETE

Breakfast—Yogurt and Fruit

Protein:	1½ cups plain low-fat yogurt
	3 ounces lean Canadian bacon
Carbohydrate:	1½ cups pineapple, cubed
Fat:	4 tablespoons slivered almonds

Cooking Instructions

Mix fruit with yogurt and top with slivered almonds. Cook the Canadian bacon separately.

Lunch—Grilled Chicken Salad

Protein:	6 ounces grilled chicken
Carbohydrate:	3 cups romaine lettuce
	1 cup mushrooms, sliced
	2 cups tomatoes, sliced
	1 cup onions, chopped
	1 ounce croutons
	Lemon juice to taste
	Sprinkling of garlic powder
	Dash Worcestershire sauce
	Pepper to taste
	Sprinkling of Parmesan cheese
	1 pear
	1 apple
Fat:	4 tablespoons olive oil and vinegar dressing

Cooking Instructions

Prepare the salad. Drizzle salad dressing over the salad. Squeeze the lemon over the salad. Season with garlic powder and Worcestershire sauce, and grind in fresh pepper. Toss until well combined. Place grilled chicken on top. Sprinkle with cheese. Have the pear and the apple for dessert.

Afternoon Snack

1 ounce cheese
½ apple
6 olives

Dinner—Pork Medallions and Apples

Protein:	6 ounces pork medallions or thinly sliced pork chops
Carbohydrate:	1 apple, sliced
	Rosemary to taste
	Dijon mustard to taste

1 tablespoon white wine

¼ cup water

1½ cups steamed broccoli

1 spinach salad

1 orange as dessert

Fat: 4 tablespoons olive oil and vinegar dressing

Cooking Instructions

Put pork into baking dish in a single layer. Top with apple slices, rosemary, and mustard. Pour wine and water around the pork. Bake at 450 degrees for 15 minutes. Baste pork with pan juices. Reduce heat to 350 degrees and continue cooking for 10–15 minutes or until pork is white, not pink, inside.

Late-Night Snack

1 ounce soft cheese

4 ounces red wine

DAY FIVE FOR THE TYPICAL AMERICAN MALE OLYMPIC ATHLETE

Breakfast—French Toast Sticks

Protein: 8 egg whites or 1 cup egg substitute

2 ounces lean Canadian bacon

Carbohydrate: 2 slices of whole grain bread

2 cups strawberries, sliced

Fat: 4 tablespoons slivered almonds

Cooking Instructions

Cut bread into sticks and soak in beaten eggs. (Scramble any egg mixture that remains.) Spray a nonstick pan with vegetable spray. Over medium-low heat, cook breadsticks, turning often, until done. Top with sliced strawberries and slivered almonds. Cook the Canadian bacon as a side dish.

Lunch—Chicken Salad Sandwich

Protein: 6 ounces cooked chicken
                                           breast, shredded

Carbohydrate: Celery, chopped
                                           1 cup grapes
                                           Lettuce
                                           Tomato slice
                                           2 pieces rye bread or 1 regular
                                           pita pocket

Fat: 4 tablespoons light mayonnaise

Cooking Instructions

Mix shredded chicken with mayonnaise, celery, and grapes. Put into mini pita pocket and add tomato slice and lettuce.

Afternoon Snack

1 tablespoon guacamole
                 wrapped in 1 ounce sliced
                 turkey
½ cup grapes
2 macadamia nuts

Dinner—Meatloaf

Protein: 9 ounces lean ground beef (less
                                           than 10 percent fat) or
                                           ground turkey
                                           4 tablespoons egg substitute

Carbohydrate: 1 tablespoon ketchup
                                           ¼ cup onions, chopped
                                           1 teaspoon bread crumbs
                                           Dash Worcestershire sauce
                                           Pepper to taste
                                           1½ cups cooked zucchini
                                           1 apple
                                           1 orange
                                           1 tossed salad

Fat: 4 tablespoons olive oil and
vinegar dressing

Cooking Instructions

Mix ground meat, egg substitute, ketchup, onions, bread crumbs, pepper, and Worcestershire sauce. Form into shallow loaf and place in microwave-safe dish. Cover with waxed paper. Microwave on medium for 10–15 minutes or until done. Have the apple and orange for dessert.

Late-Night Snack

1 ounce turkey breast, sliced
1 cup strawberries
1 tablespoon guacamole

DAY SIX FOR THE TYPICAL AMERICAN MALE OLYMPIC ATHLETE

Breakfast—Skillet Hash

Protein: 6 ounces cooked lean meat
(chicken, ham, or beef)
Carbohydrate: ⅔ cup cooked potato, diced
2 cups tomato, chopped
Green bell pepper, onions, and
mushrooms to taste, chopped
Salt and pepper to taste
Dash Worcestershire sauce
½ cantaloupe
Fat: 4 tablespoons olive oil

Cooking Instructions

In nonstick pan, sauté green pepper, onions, and mushrooms in olive oil until tender. Add cooked meat, potato, tomato, spices, and Worcestershire sauce. Cook, stirring, until heated through. Have cantaloupe as side dish.

Lunch—BLT Sandwich

Protein: 3 ounces cooked extra-lean
                              Canadian bacon
                            1½ ounces deli-style turkey
                              (added to salad)
                            2 ounces nonfat cheese
                            Lettuce and sliced tomato
                            ½ pear
                            1 tossed salad (see Food Block
                              guide)
Carbohydrate: 2 slices rye bread
Fat: 1 tablespoon light mayonnaise
                            3 tablespoons olive oil and
                              vinegar dressing

Afternoon Snack

                            2 ounces low-fat cottage cheese
                            ½ cup pineapple, diced
                            6 olives, sliced

Dinner—Quick Turkey Dinner

Protein: 9 ounces deli-style turkey breast
                              or 6 ounces cooked skinless
                              turkey breast
Carbohydrate: 3 cups steamed broccoli
                            ½ cup boiled and drained onions
                            ¼ cup cranberries
                            1 nectarine for dessert
Fat: 1 tablespoon slivered almonds
                            9 macadamia nuts

Late-Night Snack

                            1 ounce turkey breast, sliced
                            1 cup strawberries
                            6 almonds

DAY SEVEN FOR THE TYPICAL AMERICAN MALE
OLYMPIC ATHLETE

Breakfast—Scrambled Eggs Benedict

Protein:	2 ounces lean Canadian bacon
	8 large egg whites or 1 cup egg substitute
Carbohydrate:	1 English muffin
	½ grapefruit
	1 cup strawberries
Fat:	4 teaspoons olive oil

Cooking Instructions

Beat egg whites and olive oil with a little milk if desired. Spray a nonstick pan with vegetable spray and then scramble the eggs. Toast the English muffin. Cook the Canadian bacon, place on the toasted muffin, and top with the eggs.

Lunch—Turkey in a Pocket

Protein:	9 ounces deli-style turkey breast or 6 ounces cooked turkey breast
Carbohydrate:	1 mini pita pocket
	1 green bell pepper, chopped
	1 tomato, sliced
	1 cup strawberries
	1 orange
Fat:	6 tablespoons guacamole

Afternoon Snack

2 hard-boiled egg whites
½ apple
6 almonds

Dinner—Broiled Salmon

Protein:	9 ounces salmon fillet
Carbohydrate:	Rosemary to taste
	Tarragon to taste
	Dill to taste
	Lemon (optional)
	1½ cups cooked zucchini
	2 tomatoes, split, broiled, and sprinkled with Parmesan cheese)
	1 apple
	1 orange
Fat:	4 teaspoons olive oil
	Sprinkling of Parmesan cheese

Cooking Instructions

Rub the fillet with the herbs, and then brush with olive oil. Broil for 10 minutes per inch of thickness, turning and basting once. Garnish with lemon if desired. Have the apple and orange for dessert

Late-Night Snack

1 ounce turkey breast, sliced
1 cup strawberries
2 macadamia nuts

9

ZONE RECIPES

If Zone cooking sounds boring, or too mathematical, then this chapter might just change your mind. It contains more than one hundred and fifty great-tasting, easy-to-make meals designed by chef Scott C. Lane that all have same 1:1:1 block ratio of protein, carbohydrate, and fat that will help get you into and maintain yourself in the Zone.

Zone recipes have to look great, taste great, be easy to prepare, and be hormonally correct. You will find that these Zone recipes are a little different from most recipes in that they are laid out in eight-block segments. This means that each recipe contains eight blocks of protein, eight blocks of carbohydrate, and eight blocks of added fat. Depending on how many blocks you and your family require, simply adjust the recipe size accordingly (as explained in Chapter 8, "A Week in the Zone"). The typical adult female will require two to three blocks per meal, the typical adult male will require three to four blocks, and the typical child will require two blocks per meal. And if you're cooking for one, either cut down the size of the meal or make the entire recipe and freeze the portion you don't plan to eat. You should also note that many of the Zone lunches can also be used for dinners.

These recipes are also designed to be extremely flexible. If you want to serve a hearty salad, then simply subtract one carbohydrate block from the recipe for each salad you plan to make. If you want a glass of wine or cocktail with a meal, then further subtract the amount of alcohol in terms of carbohydrate blocks (see Appendix B for a listing) from the remaining carbohydrate blocks in that recipe. If you want a dessert, then make a further reduction in the remaining carbohydrate blocks found in each recipe. By making the appropriate carbohydrate adjustments for salads, alcohol, or desserts, you will always keep your hormonal carburetor in tune.

Because these meals contain a lot of low-density carbohydrates, like fruits and vegetables, many people will even have trouble eating the entire meal despite the fact that the calorie content of a typical four-block portion of one of the following recipes will be under 400 calories.

Don't think of these as meals, think of them as some of the most powerful drugs you will ever be prescribed. I guarantee you that after a week of Zone meals and snacks, you will never look at a bagel or plate of pasta the same way again.

BREAKFAST

Mexican Omelette

Servings: 2 omelettes (four blocks each)

Block Size:

2 Protein	2 whole eggs*
6 Protein	12 egg whites
2 Carbohydrate	2 cups onion, minced
2 Carbohydrate	½ cup cooked chickpeas
2 Carbohydrate	½ cup cooked kidney beans
⅔ Carbohydrate	1 cup green bell pepper, diced
⅔ Carbohydrate	1 cup red bell pepper, diced
⅔ Carbohydrate	2 cups mushrooms, minced
8 Fat	2⅔ teaspoons olive oil, divided

⅛ teaspoon black pepper
⅛ teaspoon hot sauce (or to taste)
⅛ teaspoon dry mustard
¼ teaspoon turmeric
⅛ teaspoon chili powder
4 garlic cloves, minced, divided

Method:
In a medium nonstick sauté pan, cook onion, garlic, chickpeas, kidney beans, red and green peppers, and mushrooms in ⅔ teaspoon oil until tender. In a mixing bowl, whip together whole eggs, egg whites, black pepper, hot sauce, mustard, turmeric, and chili powder. In a second sauté pan, heat 1 teaspoon oil before adding half the egg mixture. Cook until set and an omelette is formed. Fill omelette with half the vegetable mixture, fold over and serve. Repeat process to make second omelette.

Note: Eggs used in these recipes are sized as large.

Scrambled Vegetable Delight

Servings: 2 Scrambled Vegetable Delight Dishes (four blocks each)

Block Size:

2 Protein	2 ounces skim milk mozzarella cheese, shredded
4 Protein	8 egg whites
2 Protein	2 whole eggs*
1 Carbohydrate	2 cups broccoli, chopped
1 Carbohydrate	3 cups mushrooms, diced
2 Carbohydrate	3 cups red bell pepper, diced
2 Carbohydrate	2 cups onion, diced
1 Carbohydrate	1 cup yellow squash, diced
1 Carbohydrate	1 cup zucchini, diced
8 Fat	2⅔ teaspoons olive oil
	⅛ teaspoon nutmeg
	¼ teaspoon turmeric
	⅛ teaspoon black pepper
	⅛ teaspoon celery salt

Method:

In a medium nonstick sauté pan, cook vegetables in oil until almost tender. In a mixing bowl, combine whole eggs, egg whites, cheese, nutmeg, and turmeric. Mix egg mixture well until all ingredients are blended together. Pour egg mixture over vegetables and continue cooking while stirring. As the egg mixture starts to cook, it will resemble scrambled eggs. When Scrambled Vegetable Delight is cooked to your liking, divide and place on two warmed serving plates. Lightly sprinkle with black pepper and celery salt and serve.

Note: Eggs used in these recipes are sized as large.

Breakfast Fruit Salad

Servings: 2 Breakfast Fruit Salad dishes (four blocks each)

Block Size:

8 Protein	2 cups low-fat cottage cheese
1 Carbohydrate	½ cup maraschino cherries
1 Carbohydrate	1 cup strawberries, sliced
2 Carbohydrate	1 cup blueberries
2 Carbohydrate	2 kiwi fruit, peeled and diced
2 Carbohydrate	⅔ cup mandarin orange sections
8 Fat	24 black olives, chopped
	2 tablespoon fresh mint, diced
	⅛ teaspoon banana extract
	⅛ teaspoon parsley flakes

Method:
In a mixing bowl, combine all ingredients and gently blend. Mound on two plates, sprinkle with parsley, and serve immediately, because it does not hold up well after several hours.

Apple-Cinnamon Raisin Omelette

Servings: 2 omelettes (four blocks each)

Block Size:

6 Protein	8 egg whites plus 2 whole eggs*
2 Protein	2 envelopes Knox Unflavored Gelatin
4 Carbohydrate	2 red Delicious apples, cored and sliced
2 Carbohydrate	2 tablespoons raisins
2 Carbohydrate	⅔ cup applesauce
8 Fat	2⅔ teaspoons olive oil

½ cup water

½ teaspoon plus ⅛ teaspoon cinnamon

⅛ teaspoon turmeric

Method:
In a medium nonstick sauté pan, place apples, raisins, and water. Simmer mixture under medium heat for 3–4 minutes until apples soften slightly. In a mixing bowl, add gelatin, applesauce, ⅔ teaspoon oil, and ½ teaspoon cinnamon. Add applesauce mixture to apple-raisin mixture and mix well, simmering an additional 3–4 minutes. Place apple-applesauce mixture aside and keep warm. In a mixing bowl, whip egg whites, whole eggs, and turmeric together. Heat 1 teaspoon oil in a second sauté pan. Pour half the egg mixture into the sauté pan and cook until egg sets and an omelette forms. As the omelette is cooking, lightly sprinkle with a dash (⅛ teaspoon) of cinnamon. When omelette is cooked place half the filling on omelette and fold over. Remove to serving plate and serve immediately. Repeat process to make second omelette.

*Note: Eggs used in these recipes are sized as large.

Italian Breakfast Omelette

Servings: 2 omelettes (four blocks each)

Block Size:

6 Protein	8 egg whites plus 2 whole eggs*
2 Protein	2 ounces skim milk mozzarella cheese
2½ Carbohydrate	3½ cups cooked zucchini, sliced
1 Carbohydrate	3 cups cooked mushrooms, sliced
1½ Carbohydrate	1½ cups onion rings, halved
3 Carbohydrate	1½ cups tomato purée
8 Fat	2⅔ teaspoons olive oil, divided

⅛ teaspoon dried marjoram
⅛ teaspoon dried basil
⅛ teaspoon black pepper
⅛ teaspoon dried oregano
⅛ teaspoon turmeric

Method:
In a medium nonstick sauté pan, cook all vegetables, except tomato puree, in ⅔ teaspoon oil until almost tender. Add tomato puree, marjoram, basil, pepper, and oregano to vegetables and simmer for 3–5 minutes. Keep vegetable mixture warm. In a mixing bowl, whip egg whites, whole eggs, and turmeric together. Heat 1 teaspoon oil in a second sauté pan. Pour half the egg mixture into the sauté pan and cook until egg sets and an omelette forms. When omelette is cooked, place half the vegetable-tomato filling on omelette and fold over. Remove to serving plate, sprinkle omelette with 1 ounce mozzarella cheese and serve immediately. Repeat process to make second omelette.

*Note: Eggs used in these recipes are sized as large.

Pancakes with Strawberry Sauce

Servings: 2 dishes of pancakes (four blocks each)

Block Size:

2 Protein	2 whole eggs
4 Protein and 4 Carbohydrate	1⅓ cups soy flour*
2 Protein and 2 Carbohydrate	2 cups 1 percent milk
2 Carbohydrate	2 cups strawberries, sliced
8 Fat	2⅔ teaspoons olive oil
	3 teaspoons strawberry extract, divided**
	2 tablespoons water

Method:
In a small mixing bowl, combine eggs, soy flour, milk, and 2 teaspoons of strawberry extract to form a thin batter. Heat ⅔ teaspoon oil in a nonstick sauté pan. Pour batter into pan to make small (two-inch) pancakes. Batter will make about 24 silver dollar–sized pancakes. The pancakes will cook to a golden brown in color and will resemble buckwheat pancakes in color and flavor. As pancakes are cooked, place on two serving plates and keep warm. Repeat process until all the batter is used. When you have finished making all the pancakes, add sliced strawberries, water, and ½ teaspoon extract to the sauté pan. Lightly heat strawberries until they are warm. Place strawberry mixture on top of pancakes on both plates and serve.

Note: Available in some health food stores.

**Note: Strawberry extract is needed in the batter to give it the buckwheat taste and to moderate the strong flavor of the soy flour.*

Pancakes with Maple-Cinnamon Sauce

Servings: 2 dishes of pancakes (four blocks each)

Block Size:

2 Protein	2 whole eggs
4 Protein and 4 Carbohydrate	1⅓ cups soy flour*
2 Protein and 2 Carbohydrate	2 cups 1 percent milk
2 Carbohydrate	⅔ cup unsweetened applesauce
8 Fat	2⅔ teaspoons olive oil

2 tablespoons strawberry extract**
2 tablespoons plus ⅛ teaspoon
   maple flavor
2 tablespoons water
⅛ teaspoon cinnamon

Method:
In a small mixing bowl, combine eggs, soy flour, milk, strawberry extract, and ⅛ teaspoon maple flavor to form a thin batter. Heat ⅔ teaspoon oil in a nonstick sauté pan. Pour batter into pan to make small (two-inch) pancakes. Batter will make about 24 silver dollar–sized pancakes. The pancakes will cook to a golden brown color and will resemble buckwheat pancakes in color and flavor. As pancakes are cooked, place on two serving plates and keep warm. Repeat process until all the batter is used. When you have finished making all the pancakes, add applesauce, cinnamon, 2 tablespoons water, and 2 tablespoons maple flavor to the sauté pan. Lightly heat applesauce until warm. Place applesauce mixture on top of pancakes on both plates and serve.

Note: Available in some health food stores.

**Note: Strawberry extract is needed in batter to give it the buckwheat taste and to moderate the strong flavor of the soy flour.*

Blueberry Pancakes

Servings: 2 dishes of pancakes (four blocks each)

Block Size:

2 Protein	2 whole eggs
4 Protein and 4 Carbohydrate	1⅓ cups soy flour*
2 Protein and 2 Carbohydrate	2 cups 1 percent milk
2 Carbohydrate	1 cup blueberries
8 Fat	2 ⅔ teaspoons olive oil
	2 tablespoons strawberry extract**

Method:
In a small mixing bowl, combine eggs, soy flour, milk, strawberry extract, and blueberries to form a thin batter. Heat ⅔ teaspoon oil in a nonstick sauté pan. Pour batter into pan to make small (two-inch) pancakes. Batter will make about 24 silver dollar–sized pancakes. The pancakes will cook to a golden brown color and will resemble buckwheat pancakes in color and flavor. As blueberry pancakes are cooked, place on two serving plates and keep warm. Repeat process until all the batter is used.

Note: Available in some health food stores.

**Note: Strawberry extract is needed in batter to give it the buckwheat taste and to moderate the strong flavor the soy flour.*

Breakfast Sandwich with Cheese

Servings: 2 sandwiches (four blocks each)

Block Size:

6 Protein	8 egg whites plus 2 whole eggs*
2 Protein	2 ounces skim milk mozzarella cheese, shredded
1 Carbohydrate	2 cups celery, diced fine
2 Carbohydrate	1 cup carrots, diced fine
2 Carbohydrate	2 cups onion, diced fine
3 Carbohydrate	3 cups tomato, chopped
8 Fat	2⅔ teaspoons olive oil, divided

Salt and pepper to taste
2 garlic cloves, minced
⅛ teaspoon marjoram
⅛ teaspoon Worcestershire sauce
¼ teaspoon chives
1 teaspoon parsley
⅛ teaspoon turmeric

Method:

In a medium nonstick sauté pan, cook all vegetables and spices, except turmeric, in ⅔ teaspoon oil until almost tender. Keep vegetable mixture warm. In a mixing bowl, whip egg whites, whole eggs, and turmeric together. Heat ½ teaspoon oil in a second sauté pan. Pour a quarter of the egg mixture into the sauté pan and cook until egg sets and an omelette forms. Repeat process to make three more omelettes. When the four omelettes have been made, place one omelette on each serving plate. Spoon half the vegetable mixture onto each omelette, then place the second omelette on top of vegetable mixture to form a sandwich. Sprinkle shredded cheese on top of each breakfast sandwich and serve.

Note: Eggs used in these recipes are sized as large.

Ground Turkey Omelette Sandwich

Servings: 2 sandwiches (four blocks each)

Block Size:

2 Protein	3 ounces ground turkey
6 Protein	8 egg whites plus 2 whole eggs*
2 Carbohydrate	½ cup cooked kidney beans
2 Carbohydrate	2 cups onion, diced
2 Carbohydrate	2 cups green beans, chopped
1 Carbohydrate	1½ cups green bell pepper, chopped
1 Carbohydrate	1½ cups red bell pepper, chopped
8 Fat	2⅔ teaspoons olive oil

1 teaspoon Worcestershire sauce
½ teaspoon hot sauce
3 garlic cloves, minced
Salt and pepper to taste
⅛ teaspoon turmeric

Method:
In a medium nonstick sauté pan, cook ground turkey, vegetables, and spices, except turmeric, in ⅔ teaspoon oil until almost tender. Keep turkey-vegetable mixture warm. In a mixing bowl, whip egg whites, whole eggs, and turmeric together. Heat ½ teaspoon oil in a second sauté pan. Pour a quarter of the egg mixture into the sauté pan and cook until egg sets and an omelette forms. Repeat process to make three more omelettes. When the four omelettes have been made, place one omelette on each serving plate. Spoon half the turkey-vegetable mixture onto each omelette, then place the second omelette on top of each turkey-vegetable mixture to form a sandwich. Serve immediately.

Note: Eggs used in these recipes are sized as large.

Vegetarian Breakfast Omelette Sandwich

Servings: 2 sandwiches (four blocks each)

Block Size:

8 Protein	10 egg whites plus 2 whole eggs*
2 Carbohydrate	2 cups onion, diced
2 Carbohydrate	2 cups leeks, diced
2 Carbohydrate	1 cup carrots, diced
2 Carbohydrate	6 cups mushrooms, sliced
8 Fat	2⅔ teaspoons olive oil

1 tablespoon parsley
1 clove garlic, minced
Salt and pepper to taste
⅛ teaspoon turmeric

Method:

In a medium nonstick sauté pan, cook all vegetables and spices, except turmeric, in ⅔ teaspoon oil until almost tender. Keep vegetable mixture warm. In a mixing bowl, whip egg whites, whole eggs, and turmeric together. Heat ½ teaspoon oil in a second sauté pan. Pour a quarter of the egg mixture into the sauté pan and cook until egg sets and an omelette forms. Repeat process to make three more omelettes. When the four omelettes have been made, place one omelette on each serving plate. Spoon half the vegetable mixture onto each omelette, then place the second omelette on top of each vegetable mixture to form a sandwich. Serve immediately.

Note: Eggs used in these recipes are sized as large.

Breakfast Spinach Omelette Pie

Servings: 2 pies (four blocks each)

Block Size:

6 Protein	8 egg whites plus 2 whole eggs*
2 Protein	2 ounces skim milk mozzarella cheese
4 Carbohydrate	1 pound spinach
3½ Carbohydrate	3½ cups onion, diced fine
½ Carbohydrate	½ cup shallots, diced fine
8 Fat	2⅔ teaspoons olive oil
	⅛ teaspoon black pepper
	2 garlic cloves, minced
	½ teaspoon nutmeg
	⅛ teaspoon turmeric

Method:

In a medium nonstick sauté pan, cook all vegetables and spices, except turmeric, in ⅔ teaspoon oil until almost tender. Keep spinach mixture warm. In a mixing bowl, whip egg whites, whole eggs, and turmeric together. Heat 1 teaspoon oil in a second sauté pan. Pour half the egg mixture into the sauté pan and cook until egg sets and an omelette forms. Repeat process to make another omelette. Place omelettes in the bottom of two soup bowls. Spoon half the spinach mixture onto each omelette to form a spinach pie. Top with shredded cheese and serve.

Note: Eggs used in these recipes are sized as large.

Breakfast Zucchini Omelette Pie

Servings: 2 pies (four blocks each)

Block Size:

6 Protein	8 egg whites plus 2 whole eggs*
2 Protein	2 ounces skim milk mozzarella cheese
4 Carbohydrate	6 cups zucchini, quartered
2 Carbohydrate	2 cups onion, half ring slices
2 Carbohydrate	3 cups green bell pepper, diced
8 Fat	2⅔ teaspoons olive oil
	6 garlic cloves, minced
	2 tablespoons fresh basil, diced
	⅛ teaspoon dried oregano
	⅛ teaspoon turmeric

Method:
In a medium nonstick sauté pan, cook all vegetables and spices, except turmeric, in ⅔ teaspoon oil until almost tender. Keep zucchini mixture warm. In a mixing bowl, whip egg whites, whole eggs, and turmeric together. Heat 1 teaspoon oil in a second sauté pan. Pour half the egg mixture into the sauté pan and cook until egg sets and an omelette forms. Repeat process to make another omelette. Place omelettes in the bottom of two soup bowls. Spoon half the zucchini mixture onto each omelette to form a zucchini pie. Top with shredded cheese and serve.

Note: Eggs used in these recipes are sized as large.

Breakfast Mirepoux Omelette Soufflé

Servings: 2 soufflés (four blocks each)

Block Size:

8 Protein	12 egg whites plus 2 whole eggs*
1 Carbohydrate	½ cup carrots
2 Carbohydrate	4 cups celery, diced fine
3 Carbohydrate	3 cups onion, diced fine
1 Carbohydrate	¼ cup cooked or canned kidney beans, chopped
1 Carbohydrate	2 teaspoons granulated sugar
8 Fat	2⅔ teaspoons olive oil
	⅛ teaspoon black pepper
	⅛ teaspoon celery salt
	⅛ teaspoon dried oregano

Method:

In a medium nonstick sauté pan, cook all vegetables and spices in ⅔ teaspoon oil until almost tender. Remove from heat and cool. When vegetable mixture has cooled, add beaten whole eggs and set aside. In a mixing bowl, whip egg whites and sugar to form a meringue (a marshmallowlike consistency). Heat 1 teaspoon oil in a second sauté pan. Gently pour half the meringue mixture into pan. On medium-high heat cook meringue until it has an omelette-like look and will slide around the pan. Carefully pour half the vegetable-egg mixture into the center of meringue. Continue cooking until filling is set. Fold meringue sides onto center to form a trifold. Remove to serving plate. Cut a slice down the middle of each soufflé to reveal the filling. Repeat process to make second soufflé.

Note: Eggs used in these recipes are sized as large.

Breakfast Asparagus Omelette Soufflé

Servings: 2 soufflés (four blocks each)

Block Size:

8 Protein	12 egg whites plus 2 whole eggs*
2 Carbohydrate	2 cups onion, chopped
3 Carbohydrate	3 cups asparagus, chopped
1 Carbohydrate	2¼ cups green bell pepper, chopped
2 Carbohydrate	4 teaspoons granulated sugar
8 Fat	2⅔ teaspoons olive oil
	⅛ teaspoon dried dill weed
	⅛ teaspoon dried chives
	⅛ teaspoon hot sauce
	⅛ teaspoon celery salt

Method:

In a medium nonstick sauté pan, cook all vegetables and spices in ⅔ teaspoon oil until almost tender. Remove from heat and cool. When vegetable mixture has cooled, add beaten whole eggs and set aside. In a mixing bowl, whip egg whites and sugar to form a meringue (a marshmallowlike consistency). Heat 1 teaspoon oil in a second sauté pan. Gently pour half the meringue mixture into pan. On medium-high heat cook meringue until it has an omelette-like look and will slide around the pan. Carefully pour half the vegetable-egg mixture into the center of meringue. Continue cooking until filling is set. Fold meringue sides onto center to form a trifold. Remove to serving plate. Cut a slice down the middle of each soufflé to reveal the filling. Repeat process to make second soufflé.

Note: Eggs used in these recipes are sized as large.

Breakfast Creole Omelette Soufflé

Servings: 2 soufflés (four blocks each)

Block Size:

8 Protein	12 egg whites plus 2 whole eggs*
1 Carbohydrate	½ cup carrots
2 Carbohydrate	4 cups celery, diced fine
3 Carbohydrate	3 cups onion, diced fine
2 Carbohydrate	4 teaspoons granulated sugar
8 Fat	2⅔ teaspoons olive oil
	⅛ teaspoon black pepper
	⅛ teaspoon celery salt
	⅛ teaspoon dried oregano

Method:
In a medium nonstick sauté pan, cook all vegetables and spices in ⅔ teaspoon oil until almost tender. Remove from heat and cool. When vegetable mixture has cooled, add beaten whole eggs and set aside. In a mixing bowl, whip egg whites and sugar to form a meringue (a marshmallowlike consistency). Heat 1 teaspoon oil in a second sauté pan. Gently pour half the meringue mixture into pan. On medium-high heat cook meringue until it has an omelette-like look and will slide around the pan. Carefully pour half the vegetable-egg mixture into the center of meringue. Continue cooking until filling is set. Fold meringue sides onto center to form a trifold. Remove to serving plate. Cut a slice down the middle of each soufflé to reveal the filling. Repeat process to make second soufflé.

*Note: Eggs used in these recipes are sized as large.

Apple-Cinnamon Crepe

Servings: 2 dishes of crepes (four blocks each)

Block Size:

2 Protein	2 whole eggs
4 Protein	6 ounces deli ham, diced fine
1 Protein and 1 Carbohydrate	⅓ cup soy flour*
1 Protein and 1 Carbohydrate	1 cup 1 percent milk
2 Carbohydrate	2 red Delicious apples, peeled, cored, and roughly chopped
2 Carbohydrate	⅔ cup applesauce
2 Carbohydrate	⅔ cup cooked oatmeal
8 Fat	2⅔ teaspoons olive oil
	¼ teaspoon cinnamon

Method:

In a small mixing bowl, combine eggs, soy flour, and milk to form a batter. This amount of batter will make four crepes. Pour ½ teaspoon oil into a nonstick sauté pan or crepe pan. When the oil is hot add a quarter of the batter to pan. Cover pan with another sauté or crepe pan. Cook on medium-high heat until bottom is set and crepe will move easily in pan. To turn crepe over, securely place second pan over first and turn pan over. The crepe will then be in the second sauté pan. The second side of the crepe should cook for only a minute or so to color it. Transfer crepe to serving plate and repeat process to make three more crepes. (If you need more oil in the crepe pan, omit oil from crepe filling and use it for cooking the crepes.) Place apples, applesauce, oatmeal, ⅔ teaspoon oil, ham, and cinnamon in another sauté pan to form crepe filling. Using low heat, cook mixture until apples are tender. When ready, divide filling among the four crepes by placing it in a line along the center of each crepe. Fold over the sides to make a trifold. Serve immediately, two crepes per plate.

*Note: Available in some health food stores.

Two-Berry Crepe

Servings: 2 dishes of crepes (four blocks each)

Block Size:

2 Protein	2 whole eggs
4 Protein	1 cup low-fat cottage cheese
1 Protein and 1 Carbohydrate	⅓ cup soy flour*
1 Protein and 1 Carbohydrate	1 cup 1 percent milk
3 Carbohydrate	1½ cups blueberries
2 Carbohydrate	2 cups raspberries
1 Carbohydrate	4 teaspoons cornstarch
8 Fat	2⅔ teaspoons olive oil
	1 tablespoon orange extract
	¾ cup water

Method:
In a small mixing bowl, combine eggs, soy flour, and milk to form a batter. This amount of batter will make four crepes. Pour ½ teaspoon oil into a nonstick sauté pan or crepe pan. When the oil is hot, add a quarter of the batter to pan. Cover pan with another sauté or crepe pan. Cook on medium-high heat until bottom is set and crepe will move easily in pan. To turn crepe over, securely place second pan over first and turn pan over. The crepe will then be in the second sauté pan. The second side of the crepe should cook for only a minute or so to color it. Transfer crepe to serving plate and repeat process to make three more crepes. (If you need more oil in the crepe pan, omit oil from crepe filling and use it for cooking the crepes.) In a small bowl, add the cornstarch, orange extract, ⅔ teaspoon oil, and water until cornstarch has dissolved. While the crepes are cooking, place dissolved cornstarch in another nonstick sauté pan to make crepe filling. While stirring constantly, heat dissolved cornstarch until a sauce forms, then add berries and heat

through to create filling. When ready, divide filling among the four crepes by placing it in a line along the center of each crepe. Place ¼ cup of cottage cheese on top of filling and fold over the sides to make a trifold. Serve immediately, two crepes per plate.

Note: Available in some health food stores.

Mandarin Orange Crepe

Servings: 2 dishes of crepes (four blocks each)

Block Size:

2 Protein	2 whole eggs
1 Protein and 1 Carbohydrate	⅓ cup soy flour*
1 Protein and 1 Carbohydrate	1 cup 1 percent milk
2 Protein and 2 Carbohydrate	1 cup plain low-fat yogurt
2 Protein	2 envelopes Knox Unflavored Gelatin
1 Carbohydrate	4 teaspoons cornstarch
3 Carbohydrate	1 cup mandarin orange sections
8 Fat	2⅔ teaspoons olive oil
	2 teaspoon orange extract

Method:

In a small mixing bowl, combine eggs, soy flour, and milk to form a batter. This amount of batter will make four crepes. Pour ½ teaspoon oil into a nonstick sauté pan or crepe pan. When the oil is hot, add a quarter of the batter to pan. Cover pan with another sauté or crepe pan. Cook on medium-high heat until bottom is set and crepe will move easily in pan. To turn crepe over, securely place second pan over first and turn pan over. The crepe will then be in the second sauté pan. The second side of the crepe should cook for only a minute or so to color it. Transfer crepe to serving plate and repeat process to make three more crepes. (If you need more oil in the crepe pan, omit oil from crepe filling and use it for cooking the crepes.) In a small bowl, stir together the yogurt, cornstarch, orange extract, ⅔ teaspoon oil, and gelatin. Transfer mixture to another sauté pan to make crepe filling. Heat mixture on low heat while stirring constantly until heated throughout, then add orange sections and heat through. When ready, divide filling among the four crepes by placing it in a line along the center of each crepe. Fold over the sides to make a trifold. Serve immediately, two crepes per plate.

Note: Available in some health food stores.

Kiwi and Pineapple Crepe

Servings: 2 dishes of crepes (four blocks each)

Block Size:

2 Protein	2 whole eggs
4 Protein	1 cup low-fat cottage cheese
1 Protein and 1 Carbohydrate	⅓ cup soy flour*
1 Protein and 1 Carbohydrate	1 cup 1 percent milk
2 Carbohydrate	2 kiwi fruit, peeled and diced
4 Carbohydrate	2 cups pineapple
8 Fat	2⅔ teaspoons olive oil
	⅛ teaspoon cinnamon

Method:
In a small mixing bowl, combine eggs, soy flour, and milk to form a batter. This amount of batter will make four crepes. Pour ½ teaspoon oil into nonstick sauté pan or crepe pan. When the oil is hot

add a quarter of the batter to pan. Cover pan with another sauté or crepe pan. Cook on medium-high heat until bottom is set and crepe will move easily in pan. To turn crepe over, securely place second pan over first and turn pan over. The crepe will then be in the second sauté pan. The second side of the crepe should cook for only a minute or so to color it. Transfer crepe to serving plate and repeat process to make three more crepes. (If you need more oil in the crepe pan, omit oil from crepe filling and use it for cooking the crepes.) In a sauté pan, combine kiwi fruit, pineapple, ⅔ teaspoon oil, and cinnamon, and heat until they are tender. When the fruit is hot, divide the filling among the four crepes by placing it in a line along the center of each crepe. Place ¼ cup cottage cheese on top of filling in each crepe and fold over the sides to make a trifold. Serve immediately, two crepes per plate.

Note: Available in some health food stores.

Vegetable Breakfast Crepe

Servings: 2 dishes of crepes (four blocks each)

Block Size:

2 Protein	2 whole eggs
4 Protein	4 ounces skim milk mozzarella cheese, shredded
1 Protein and 1 Carbohydrate	⅓ cup soy flour*
1 Protein and 1 Carbohydrate	1 cup 1 percent milk
1 Carbohydrate	4 teaspoons cornstarch
1 Carbohydrate	2 cups broccoli spears, sliced thin
1 Carbohydrate	3 cups mushrooms, diced fine
1 Carbohydrate	1 cup onion, diced fine
2 Carbohydrate	2 cups strawberries, sliced
8 Fat	2 ⅔ teaspoons olive oil
	¼ teaspoon turmeric
	2 tablespoons water
	⅛ teaspoon sherry

Method:

In a small mixing bowl, combine eggs, soy flour, and milk to form a batter. This amount of batter will make four crepes. Pour ½ teaspoon oil into nonstick sauté pan or crepe pan. When the oil is hot, add a quarter of the batter to pan. Cover pan with another sauté or crepe pan. Cook on medium-high heat until bottom is set and crepe will move easily in pan. To turn crepe over, securely place second pan over first and turn pan over. The crepe will then be in the second sauté pan. The second side of the crepe should cook for only a minute or so to color it. Transfer crepe to serving plate and repeat process to make three more crepes. (If you need more oil in the crepe pan, omit oil from crepe filling and use it for cooking the crepes.) In a small saucepan combine turmeric, cornstarch, 2 tablespoons water, and sherry, and mix well. Add cheese and heat. Stir sauce continuously over moderate heat until a thick cheese sauce forms. Remove from heat and keep warm. In a sauté pan, add ⅔ teaspoon oil and cook broccoli, mushrooms, and onions until tender. When the vegetable mixture is cooked, divide the filling among the four crepes by placing it in a line along the center of each crepe. Fold over the sides to make a trifold. Serve two crepes per plate and top crepes with a small quantity of cheese sauce. Garnish each plate with 1 cup sliced strawberries beside crepe.

Note: Available in some health food stores.

Note: Can also be used as a light brunch dish.

Fresh Fruit with Creamy Sauce

Servings: 2 dishes of fruit and sauce (four blocks each)

Block Size:

8 Protein	2 cups low-fat cottage cheese
1 Carbohydrate	⅓ cup applesauce
2 Carbohydrate	2 peaches
1 Carbohydrate	½ cup grapes
1 Carbohydrate	⅓ cup mandarin orange sections
1 Carbohydrate	1 cup strawberries, sliced
2 Carbohydrate	1 apple, cored and sliced
8 Fat	8 teaspoons almonds, sliced
	¼ teaspoon cinnamon
	⅛ teaspoon nutmeg

Method:
Combine cottage cheese, cinnamon, and nutmeg in a blender. Blend until smooth. Remove from blender and place in a small mixing bowl, then add fruit and gently blend together. Divide fruit mixture into two serving dishes, top with almonds, and serve.

Sweet and Spicy Peaches

Servings: 2 dishes of peaches (four blocks each)

Block Size:

2 Protein	2 envelopes Knox Unflavored Gelatin
4 Protein	2 ounces protein powder (28 grams of protein)
2 Protein and 2 Carbohydrate	1 cup plain low-fat yogurt, lightly heated
5 Carbohydrate	5 peaches, peeled, pitted, and sliced
1 Carbohydrate	1½ teaspoons brown sugar
8 Fat	8 teaspoons almonds, sliced
	1 tablespoon vanilla extract
	⅛ teaspoon allspice
	½ cup water

Method:
In saucepan gently heat peaches, vanilla extract, allspice, brown sugar, gelatin, and water until hot. In a mixing bowl, combine protein powder with yogurt. Place yogurt and protein powder mixture and into two serving bowls, then top with heated fruit and serve.

Strawberry Instant Breakfast

Servings: 2 glasses (four blocks each)

Block Size:

2 Protein	2 envelopes Knox Unflavored Gelatin
2 Protein	½ cup low-fat cottage cheese
2 Protein and 2 Carbohydrate	2 cups 1 percent milk
2 Protein and 2 Carbohydrate	1 cup plain low-fat yogurt
4 Carbohydrate	4 cups strawberries, sliced*
8 Fat	2⅔ teaspoons olive oil

Method:
Place all ingredients in blender to make instant breakfast. Blend until smooth. Pour into two large glasses, garnish with a strawberry, and serve.

*Note: Fresh or frozen strawberries can be used. If using frozen strawberries, use whole or sliced berries without sugar or additives. If using fresh strawberries, use only those that are plump and have a solid color. Always store fresh strawberries covered in the refrigerator.

Scrambled Eggs with Vegetables

Servings: 2 scrambled egg dishes (four blocks each)

Block Size:

8 Protein	12 egg whites plus 2 whole eggs
1 Carbohydrate	4 cups spinach
2 Carbohydrate	2 cups green beans
2 Carbohydrate	2 cups wax beans
2 Carbohydrate	½ cup kidney beans
1 Carbohydrate	1 cup onion, chopped
8 Fat	2⅔ teaspoons olive oil, divided
	¼ teaspoon turmeric

Method:
In a medium nonstick sauté pan, add ⅔ teaspoon oil and all vegetables. Cook vegetables until tender, then remove from stove and keep vegetable mixture warm until scrambled eggs are made. In a mixing bowl, whip egg whites, whole eggs, and turmeric together. Heat 2 teaspoons oil in a second sauté pan. Pour the egg mixture into the sauté pan and stir continuously until scrambled eggs are cooked. Divide the scrambled eggs between two heated serving plates and place an equal amount of vegetables beside scrambled eggs.

Breakfast Pizza Omelette

Servings: 2 pizzas (four blocks each)

Block Size:

6 Protein	8 egg whites plus 2 whole eggs
2 Protein	2 ounces skim milk mozzarella cheese, shredded
1 Carbohydrate	3 cups mushrooms, sliced
1 Carbohydrate	1 cup tomato, diced
1 Carbohydrate	1 cup onion, chopped
2 Carbohydrate	½ cup chickpeas, chopped
1 Carbohydrate	1 cup asparagus, chopped
2 Carbohydrate	1 cup tomato puree
8 Fat	2⅔ teaspoons olive oil, divided
	¼ teaspoon turmeric

Method:

In a nonstick medium sauté pan, add 2 teaspoons oil and all vegetables, except tomato puree. Cook vegetables until tender, then remove from stove and keep vegetable mixture warm. In a mixing bowl, whip egg whites, whole eggs, and turmeric together. Heat ⅔ teaspoon oil in a second sauté pan, until almost hot. Pour egg mixture into second sauté pan and cook mixture until egg sets and an omelette forms. Place omelette in baking dish and spoon vegetable mixture on top, to form a topping. Heat tomato puree in small saucepan and pour over contents of baking dish. Top with shredded cheese and place under broiler until cheese melts and browns slightly. Cut into four wedges and serve two wedges per serving plate.

Sausage and Egg Breakfast with Vegetables

Servings: 2 Sausage and Egg Breakfast dishes (four blocks each)

Block Size:

6 Protein	9 ounces ground turkey
2 Protein	2 whole eggs
2 Carbohydrate	2 cups kale
1 Carbohydrate	1 cup leeks, sliced
1 Carbohydrate	2 cups steamed broccoli florets
1 Carbohydrate	½ cup steamed carrots, half slices
1 Carbohydrate	¾ cup red bell pepper, half rings
1 Carbohydrate	1 cup steamed wax beans, chopped
1 Carbohydrate	½ apple, shredded
8 Fat	2⅔ teaspoons olive oil, divided

⅛ teaspoon sage
⅛ teaspoon paprika
⅛ teaspoon nutmeg
Salt and pepper to taste
Water

Method:
In a saucepan, add vegetables with enough water to cover vegetables. Cook vegetables until tender but not overcooked. In a mixing bowl, combine turkey, apple, sage, paprika, nutmeg, salt, and pepper. Form turkey mixture into two patties and sauté in ⅔ teaspoon oil. Remove patties from pan and set aside. In a nonstick sauté pan, heat 2 teaspoons oil, then cook whole eggs over easy. Place vegetables on two plates along with a turkey sausage patty and an over-easy egg on each plate.

Omelette à la Colorado

Servings: 2 omelettes (four blocks each)

Block Size:

6 Protein	8 egg whites plus 2 eggs
1 Protein	1½ ounces deli-style ham, chopped
1 Protein	1 ounce skim milk mozzarella cheese, shredded
1 Carbohydrate	1 cup onion, diced fine
2 Carbohydrate	2 cups kale
1 Carbohydrate	¼ cup cooked black beans
1 Carbohydrate	¼ cup cooked kidney beans
1 Carbohydrate	¼ cup cooked chickpeas
1 Carbohydrate	1 cup onion, chopped fine
½ Carbohydrate	¾ cup green bell pepper, chopped
½ Carbohydrate	¾ cup red bell pepper, chopped
8 Fat	2⅔ teaspoons olive oil

Method:

In a medium nonstick sauté pan, cook 1 cup diced fine onion, kale, beans, and chickpeas in ⅔ teaspoon oil until hot and crisp. In a mixing bowl, whip together whole eggs, egg whites, chopped peppers, 1 cup chopped fine onions, ham, and cheese. In a second sauté pan, heat 1 teaspoon oil before adding half the egg mixture. Cook until set and an omelette is formed. Repeat process to make second omelette. Fill each omelette with half the vegetable mixture, then fold over and serve.

Eggs Arnold

Servings: 2 egg dishes (four blocks each)

Block Size:

4 Protein	4 egg whites plus 2 whole eggs, separated
2 Protein	2 ounces skim milk mozzarella cheese, shredded
2 Protein	3 ounces deli-style ham
1½ Carbohydrate	4 Portobello mushroom caps*
1 Carbohydrate	¾ cup red bell pepper, thin strips
2 Carbohydrate	½ cup cooked kidney beans
3 Carbohydrate	3 cups asparagus, chopped
½ Carbohydrate	2 teaspoons cornstarch
8 Fat	2⅔ teaspoons olive oil

3 tablespoons water
Dash white wine
¼ teaspoon chili powder
⅛ teaspoon turmeric

Method:
Remove stems from mushrooms, then lightly cook mushroom caps in ⅔ teaspoon oil, 1 tablespoon water, and dash white wine. Using an egg poacher, poach eggs and egg whites separately, then reserve for use. In nonstick sauté pan, cook pepper and kidney beans in 2 teaspoons oil until tender. In a saucepan, add asparagus and enough water to cover. Cook asparagus until tender but not over-cooked. In another small saucepan, combine chili powder, turmeric, cornstarch, and 2 tablespoons water. Blend mixture until cornstarch dissolves, then add mozzarella cheese and heat until a sauce forms. Assemble dish by placing two mushroom caps on each serving plate and topping mushrooms with the poached egg whites. Layer ham over mushroom capped egg white on each plate. Place a poached whole egg beside the two mushroom caps on each plate,

then gently pour sauce on top. Divide vegetables in half and place beside eggs on plates.

Note: Portobello mushrooms are large-capped mushrooms with a mild meaty flavor, which work excellently with this recipe. The mushroom stems can be diced and added to the asparagus, or saved for another dish.

Poached Eggs on a Spinach Bed

Servings: 2 egg dishes (four blocks each)

Block Size:

6 Protein	8 egg whites plus 2 whole eggs
1 Protein	¼ cup cottage cheese
1 Protein and 1 Carbohydrate	1 cup 1 percent milk
1 Carbohydrate	3 cups mushrooms, diced fine
2 Carbohydrate	2 cups onion, diced fine
2 Carbohydrate	8 cups spinach
2 Carbohydrate	4 teaspoons cornstarch
8 Fat	2⅔ teaspoons olive oil
	¼ teaspoon nutmeg
	⅛ teaspoon allspice
	⅛ teaspoon chili powder
	⅛ teaspoon paprika

Method:
Using an egg poacher, poach eggs and egg whites separately, then reserve for use. In nonstick sauté pan, cook mushrooms and onions in 2 teaspoons oil until tender, then remove and keep warm. In another sauté pan, add the remaining ⅔ teaspoon oil and cook the spinach until just wilted. Combine cottage cheese, nutmeg, allspice, chili powder, milk, and cornstarch in a blender. Blend until smooth. Remove from blender and place in a small saucepan on medium

heat until a sauce forms. Assemble dishes by forming a bed of spinach on each serving plate. Place half the onion and mushroom mixture on each dish, then place four poached egg whites and 1 poached egg on each dish. Evenly divide sauce by pouring over eggs on each serving plate. Sprinkle with paprika and serve.

Quiche Lorraine

Servings: 2 quiche (four blocks each)

Block Size:

4 Protein	4 egg whites plus 2 whole eggs
1 Protein	1½ ounces deli-style ham, shredded
2 Protein	2 ounces skim milk mozzarella cheese, shredded
1 Protein and 1 Carbohydrate	1 cup 1 percent milk
½ Carbohydrate	½ cup onion, diced fine
2 Carbohydrate	2 cups kale
1 Carbohydrate	1 cup zucchini, diced fine
1 Carbohydrate	1 cup yellow squash, diced fine
1 Carbohydrate	1 cup leeks, diced fine
½ Carbohydrate	¾ cup red bell pepper, diced fine
1 Carbohydrate	1 cup tomato, chopped
8 Fat	2⅔ teaspoons, olive oil
	⅛ teaspoon dry mustard
	⅛ teaspoon black pepper

Method:
In a nonstick sauté pan, cook all vegetables and spices in oil until tender. Let vegetables cool to room temperature. In a mixing bowl, whip together eggs and milk, then add cooled vegetables, ham, and cheese. Place combined ingredients in two circular baking dishes. Bake at 400 degrees for 45–60 minutes, serve immediately when removed from oven.

Asparagus Quiche

Servings: 2 quiches (four blocks each)

Block Size:

5 Protein	6 egg whites plus 2 whole eggs
2 Protein	2 ounces skim milk mozzarella cheese, shredded
1 Protein and 1 Carbohydrate	1 cup 1 percent milk
½ Carbohydrate	½ cup onion, diced fine
2 Carbohydrate	2 cups asparagus, sliced
2 Carbohydrate	2 cups kale
½ Carbohydrate	1½ cups mushrooms, sliced
1 Carbohydrate	½ cup carrots, sliced
1 Carbohydrate	1 cup tomato, chopped
8 Fat	2⅔ teaspoons olive oil
	Salt and pepper to taste
	2 garlic cloves, minced
	⅛ teaspoon chili powder
	⅛ teaspoon dried basil
	¼ teaspoon dried dill

Method:

In nonstick sauté pan, cook all vegetables and spices in oil until tender. Let vegetables cool to room temperature. In a mixing bowl, whip together eggs and milk, then add cooled vegetables and cheese. Place combined ingredients in two circular baking dishes. Bake at 400 degrees for 45–60 minutes, serve immediately when removed from oven.

Vegetable Quiche

Servings: 2 quiches (four blocks each)

Block Size:

5 Protein	6 egg whites plus 2 whole eggs
2 Protein	2 ounces skim milk mozzarella cheese, shredded
1 Protein and 1 Carbohydrate	1 cup 1 percent milk
½ Carbohydrate	½ cup onion, diced fine
1 Carbohydrate	4 cups spinach, stems removed
½ Carbohydrate	1 cup carrots, shredded
2 Carbohydrate	2 cups snow peas
½ Carbohydrate	1½ cups cucumber, peeled, seeded, and diced fine
½ Carbohydrate	¾ cup red bell pepper, diced fine
1 Carbohydrate	1 cup yellow squash, diced fine
1 Carbohydrate	½ cup water chestnuts, chopped
8 Fat	2⅔ teaspoons olive oil
	¼ teaspoon celery salt
	⅛ teaspoon hot curry powder
	4 garlic cloves, minced

Method:
In a nonstick sauté pan, cook all vegetables and spices in oil until tender. Let vegetables cool to room temperature. In a mixing bowl, whip together eggs and milk, then add cooled vegetables and cheese. Place combined ingredients in two circular baking dishes. Bake at 400 degrees for 45–60 minutes, serve immediately when removed from oven.

Tuesday Omelette

Servings: 2 omelettes (four blocks each)

Block Size:

1½ Protein	2¼ ounces deli-style ham, medium dice
6 Protein	12 egg whites
½ Protein and ½ Carbohydrate	¼ cup plain low-fat yogurt
1 Carbohydrate	1 cup onion, chopped
1 Carbohydrate	1¼ cups spinach, cooked
1 Carbohydrate	1¼ cups tomato, chopped
½ Carbohydrate	1 cup celery, chopped
2 Carbohydrate	1 apple, cored and sliced
2 Carbohydrate	1 cup honeydew melon, cubed
8 Fat	2⅔ teaspoons olive oil, divided

Salt and pepper to taste
¼ teaspoon turmeric
¼ teaspoon dried chives
⅛ teaspoon celery salt
⅛ teaspoon chili powder

Method:
In nonstick sauté pan, heat ham, onion, spinach, tomato, and celery in ⅔ teaspoon oil until vegetables are tender. While vegetables are cooking, in a medium mixing bowl combine egg whites, yogurt, and spices. The yogurt will appear curdled when mixed with the egg whites but it is fine. Whip the egg white–yogurt mixture until the yogurt has blended into the mixture and it no longer looks curdled. In a second nonstick sauté pan, heat 1 teaspoon oil before adding half the egg mixture. Cook until set and an omelette is formed. Fill omelette with half vegetable mixture, fold over, and serve with half the fruit arranged around the omelette. Repeat process to make second omelette.

Omelette à la California

Servings: 2 omelettes (four blocks each)

Block Size:

7½ Protein	15 egg whites
½ Protein and ½ Carbohydrate	¼ cup plain low-fat yogurt
1 Carbohydrate	⅓ cup cooked pinto beans, rinsed
1 Carbohydrate	¼ cup cooked black beans, rinsed
1 Carbohydrate	¼ cup cooked kidney beans, rinsed
1 Carbohydrate	1¼ cups tomato, chopped
1 Carbohydrate	1 cup onion, chopped
1 Carbohydrate	1 cup asparagus spears, half-inch pieces
½ Carbohydrate	3 cups spinach
1 Carbohydrate	¼ cup chickpeas
8 Fat	2⅔ teaspoons olive oil, divided
	¼ teaspoon dried dill
	Salt and pepper to taste
	¼ teaspoon dried chives
	¼ teaspoon turmeric
	⅛ teaspoon chili powder
	⅛ teaspoon celery salt

Method:
In nonstick sauté pan, heat beans, tomato, onion, asparagus, spinach, chickpeas, and dill in ⅔ teaspoon oil until vegetables are tender. While the vegetables are cooking, in a medium mixing bowl combine the egg whites, yogurt, and remaining spices. The yogurt will appear curdled when mixed with the egg whites but it is fine. Whip the egg white–yogurt mixture until the yogurt has blended into the mixture and it no longer looks curdled. In a second non-stick sauté pan, heat 1 teaspoon oil before adding half the egg mixture. Cook until set and an omelette is formed. Fill omelette with half the vegetable mixture, fold over, and serve. Repeat process to make second omelette.

LUNCH

Buddhist Vegetable Entrée

Servings: 2 lunch entrées (four blocks each)

Block Size:

8 Protein	24 ounces firm tofu, half-inch dice*
1 Carbohydrate	2½ cups celery, sliced
1 Carbohydrate	1 cup onion, sliced thin
1 Carbohydrate	3 cups cabbage, shredded
1 Carbohydrate	3 cups mushrooms, sliced thin
1 Carbohydrate	1½ cup zucchini, quartered and sliced
1 Carbohydrate	1½ cups bell pepper, sliced thin
1 Carbohydrate	3 cups bean sprouts
1 Carbohydrate	4 teaspoons cornstarch
8 Fat	2⅔ teaspoons olive oil

1 cup cold water
2 tablespoons low-sodium soy sauce
¼ teaspoon hot curry powder
½ teaspoon chili powder
Dash garlic powder
Salt and pepper to taste

Method:

In nonstick sauté pan, cook vegetables in oil until almost tender, then add ½ cup water and cover to steam sauté. In saucepan, add cold water, soy sauce, curry powder, chili powder, garlic powder, and cornstarch to form a sauce. (Mix cornstarch with a little water to dissolve it before adding to saucepan.) Heat sauce to a light simmer while constantly stirring, then add diced tofu to sauce and heat through. Add sauce and tofu to vegetables, stir, and simmer for 2–3 minutes. Divide between two lunch plates and serve at once.

*Note: Tofu has a high water content. To eliminate some of the excess water, place the blocks of tofu in a shallow dish and let stand for half an hour.

Spicy Vegetarian Tofu Primavera

Servings: 2 lunch entrées (four blocks each)

Block Size:

8 Protein	24 ounces extra-firm tofu, cubed*
1 Carbohydrate	½ cup carrots, sliced
1 Carbohydrate	1 cup onion, sliced
2 Carbohydrate	4½ cups green bell pepper, sliced
1 Carbohydrate	3 cups cabbage, shredded
2 Carbohydrate	2½ cups tomato, diced
1 Carbohydrate	4 teaspoons cornstarch
8 Fat	2⅔ teaspoons olive oil

1 cup cold water
1½ cups cold water
2 tablespoons soy sauce
⅛ teaspoon cayenne pepper
⅛ teaspoon crushed red pepper
2 garlic cloves, minced
Salt and pepper to taste

Method:
In nonstick sauté pan, cook vegetables in oil until almost tender, then add ½ cup water and cover to steam sauté. In saucepan, add cold water, soy sauce, cayenne pepper, crushed red pepper, garlic, and cornstarch to form a sauce. (Mix cornstarch with a little water to dissolve it before adding to saucepan.) Heat sauce to a light simmer, constantly stirring. Add diced tofu to sauce and heat through. Add tofu and sauce to vegetables, stir and simmer for 2–3 minutes. Divide between two lunch plates and serve at once.

*Note: Tofu has a high water content. To eliminate some of the excess water, place the blocks of tofu in a shallow dish and let stand for half an hour.

Rich and Hearty Cucumber Stew

Servings: 2 lunch entrées (four blocks each)

Block Size:

6 Protein	6 ounces skim milk mozzarella cheese, shredded
2 Protein	2 hard-boiled eggs, sliced
2 Carbohydrate	1 cup tomato puree
1 Carbohydrate	1¼ cups tomato, diced
2 Carbohydrate	6 cups cucumbers, diced
1 Carbohydrate	1½ cups green bell pepper, sliced and quartered
2 Carbohydrate	2 cups onion, diced
8 Fat	24 black olives, sliced

1 clove garlic, minced
White pepper to taste
Dash celery salt
¼ teaspoon salt
1½ teaspoons hot sauce
¼ teaspoon dry dill weed
1 cup water

Method:
Combine all ingredients except cheese and eggs in a large saucepan and bring to a boil. Cover and simmer on medium-high heat for 20–25 minutes, stirring frequently. Just before serving stew, stir in shredded mozzarella cheese, then divide into two soup bowls and garnish with egg slices.

Vegetarian Chili

Servings: 2 lunch entrées (four blocks each)

Block Size:

8 Protein	24 ounces extra-firm tofu, shredded
4 Carbohydrate	1 cup cooked kidney beans*
1 Carbohydrate	1 cup medium onion, diced
½ Carbohydrate	1 cup medium celery, diced
1½ Carbohydrate	1½ cups canned tomato, diced with juice
1 Carbohydrate	½ cup tomato puree
8 Fat	2⅔ teaspoons olive oil

1 cup water
6 garlic cloves, minced
1 teaspoon fresh basil
½ teaspoon hot sauce
4 tablespoons chili powder (or to taste)
Salt and pepper to taste

Method:
In saucepan, heat beans, onion, and celery in oil until tender, then add diced tomato, water, tomato puree, tofu, and spices. Heat entire mixture through until hot. Place an equal amount in two soup bowls and serve.

Note: When using canned beans, always rinse them off before using.

Mexican Black Bean Stew

Servings: 2 lunch entrées (four blocks each)

Block Size:

8 Protein	8 ounces skinless chicken breast, diced fine
4 Carbohydrate	1 cup cooked black beans*
½ Carbohydrate	½ cup onion, diced
½ Carbohydrate	¾ cup zucchini, diced
2 Carbohydrate	1 cup tomato puree
1 Carbohydrate	½ cup salsa
8 Fat	2⅔ teaspoons olive oil, divided
	⅔ cup water
	Salt and pepper to taste
	2 tablespoons parsley

Method:

In saucepan, heat beans, onion, and zucchini in 2 teaspoons oil until tender, then add tomato puree, water, parsley, and salsa. Continue cooking until entire mixture is hot. While the vegetables are cooking, in a sauté pan heat ⅔ teaspoon oil and stir-fry chicken until cooked. Add chicken to vegetables and simmer for 5 minutes. Place an equal amount in two soup bowls and serve.

*Note: When using canned beans, always rinse them off before using.

Beef Stir-Fry

Servings: 2 lunch entrées (four blocks each)

Block Size:

8 Protein   8 ounces beef eye of round, one-eighth-inch slices, cut in half-inch pieces

2 Carbohydrate   ½ cup cooked kidney beans
2 Carbohydrate   2 cups green beans, chopped
1 Carbohydrate   1 cup onion, diced
1 Carbohydrate   2¼ cups red bell pepper, diced
2 Carbohydrate   1 cup tomato puree

8 Fat   ⅔ teaspoons olive oil

1 teaspoon Worcestershire sauce
½ teaspoon hot sauce
4 garlic cloves, minced
1 cup beef stock
Salt and pepper to taste

Method:
In nonstick sauté pan place ⅔ teaspoon oil and beef. Cook beef until browned and done. While beef is cooking, in another sauté pan place 2 teaspoons oil, kidney beans, green beans, onion, bell pepper, Worcestershire sauce, hot sauce, and garlic. Cook until entire mixture is hot, then add tomato puree, beef stock, and cooked beef. Cook for 5 minutes until entire stir-fry is hot. Place an equal amount on two lunch plates and serve.

Herbed Beef and Bean Stew

Servings: 2 lunch entrées (four blocks each)

Block Size:

8 Protein	8 ounces beef eye of round, one-eighth-inch slices, diced
4 Carbohydrate	1 cup cooked kidney beans*
1 Carbohydrate	1 cup onion, diced
1 Carbohydrate	½ cup tomato puree
2 Carbohydrate	1 cup salsa
8 Fat	2⅔ teaspoons olive oil, divided

⅛ teaspoon Worcestershire sauce
½ cup beef stock
½ teaspoon chili powder
⅛ teaspoon dried basil
⅛ teaspoon curry powder
⅛ teaspoon dried oregano
Salt and pepper to taste

Method:
In saucepan, cook beans and onion in 2 teaspoons oil until tender, then add tomato puree, Worcestershire sauce, beef stock, spices, and salsa. Continue cooking vegetable mixture under medium heat until hot. While the vegetables are cooking, in nonstick sauté pan add remaining oil and stir-fry beef until cooked. Add beef to vegetables and simmer for 5 minutes. Place an equal amount in two soup bowls and serve.

Note: When using canned beans, always rinse them off before using.

Sweet and Sour Tofu

Servings: 2 lunch entrées (four blocks each)

Block Size:

8 Protein	24 ounces extra-firm tofu, cubed
1 Carbohydrate	2 teaspoons sugar
1 Carbohydrate	½ cup tomato puree
1 Carbohydrate	4 teaspoons cornstarch
1 Carbohydrate	½ cup pineapple, diced
4 Carbohydrate	2 cups fruit cocktail (packed in water)
8 Fat	2⅔ teaspoons olive oil
	1 cup water
	6 tablespoons vinegar
	4 tablespoons soy sauce
	⅛ teaspoon banana extract (optional)
	Salt and pepper to taste

Method:

In nonstick sauté pan, heat oil until hot, then add tofu. Cook tofu until browned on all sides. While tofu is cooking under medium heat, in saucepan add water, vinegar, sugar, tomato puree, soy sauce, banana extract, and cornstarch. (Mix cornstarch with a little water so that it is dissolved before being added to saucepan.) Cook over medium heat to form a sauce, stirring constantly. When a sauce has formed, add pineapple and fruit cocktail. Taste sauce; if sauce has too strong a vinegar taste, continue simmering for a few more minutes. The flavor will develop into a sweet and sour sauce as it cooks. Heat until fruit is hot, then add entire mixture to tofu in sauté pan. Simmer for 5 minutes, gently stirring mixture. Spoon onto two lunch dishes and serve immediately.

Chicken Stir-Fry

Servings: 2 lunch entrées (four blocks each)

Block Size:

8 Protein	8 ounces chicken tenderloins (or skinless chicken breast), cut into one-inch pieces
⅔ Carbohydrate	1½ cups red bell pepper, one-inch squares
⅔ Carbohydrate	1½ cups green bell pepper, one-inch squares
⅔ Carbohydrate	1½ cups yellow bell pepper, one-inch squares
2 Carbohydrate	3 cups broccoli florets, or diced fine
1 Carbohydrate	3 cups mushrooms, sliced
2 Carbohydrate	2½ cups tomato, diced fine
1 Carbohydrate	4 teaspoons cornstarch
8 Fat	2⅔ teaspoons olive oil
	2 tablespoons cider vinegar
	⅛ teaspoon dried basil
	⅛ teaspoon dried oregano
	Salt and pepper to taste
	2 cloves garlic, minced
	1 cup chicken stock

Method:

In nonstick sauté pan, place ⅔ teaspoon oil and chicken. Cook chicken until browned and done. While the chicken is cooking under medium heat, in another nonstick sauté pan place 2 teaspoons oil, bell peppers, broccoli, mushrooms, vinegar, garlic, tomato, and spices. Heat vegetables until entire mixture is hot, then add chicken stock, cooked chicken, and cornstarch. Mix cornstarch into chicken stock so it can dissolve before adding to pan. Cook for 5 minutes until entire stir-fry is hot and cornstarch has thickened the dish. Place an equal amount on two lunch plates and serve.

Note: When getting vegetable ingredients ready for a stir-fry dish be sure to cut vegetables as close to the same size as possible. This helps in making the cooking time the same.

Curried Chicken

Servings: 2 lunch entrées (four blocks each)

Block Size:

6 Protein	6 ounces chicken, diced
2 Protein and 2 Carbohydrate	1 cup plain low-fat yogurt
1 Carbohydrate	4 teaspoons cornstarch
2 Carbohydrate	6 cups mushrooms, sliced
1 Carbohydrate	2¼ cups red bell pepper, in strips
2 Carbohydrate	2 cups snow peas, in strips
8 Fat	2⅔ teaspoon olive oil

⅛ teaspoon white wine
½ cup chicken stock
2 teaspoons hot curry powder*
Salt and pepper to taste

Method:
In nonstick sauté pan, place ⅔ teaspoon oil and diced chicken. Cook chicken until browned and done, then add wine, chicken stock, yogurt, curry powder, and cornstarch. (Mix cornstarch in chicken stock so that it can dissolve before being added to pan.) Stirring constantly, heat until a thick curried sauce forms, then simmer for 5 minutes. While the chicken is cooking, in another sauté pan place 2 teaspoons oil, mushrooms, bell pepper, and snow peas. Cook until mixture is tender. Place an equal amount of cooked snow peas, bell pepper, and mushrooms on two lunch plates, then spoon the chicken curry mixture onto the plates.

Note: There are a number of brands of curry powder. Each has a slightly different blend of spices and level of heat. Experiment until you find one that fits your family's tastes.

Deviled Snow Peas

Servings: 2 lunch entrées (four blocks each)

Block Size:

2 Protein	6 ounces extra-firm tofu
2 Protein	2 whole eggs
4 Protein and	
4 Carbohydrate	2 cups plain low-fat yogurt
3 Carbohydrate	3 cups snow peas, whole
1 Carbohydrate	4 teaspoons cornstarch
8 Fat	2⅔ teaspoons olive oil
	4 teaspoons dry mustard
	2 garlic cloves, minced
	Paprika for garnish
	Salt and pepper to taste

Method:

In nonstick sauté pan, place oil and snow peas. Cook snow peas until tender. While the snow peas are cooking, in saucepan add yogurt, mustard, tofu, garlic, and eggs. Cook yogurt-tofu mixture over medium heat for 5–10 minutes until mixture is hot and tofu has broken down. (Mix cornstarch with a little water, then add to saucepan.) Stirring constantly, heat until a thick sauce forms, then add cooked snow peas. Continue simmering for 2–3 minutes. Place an equal amount of the deviled snow peas on two lunch plates, then sprinkle with paprika and serve.

Creamy Dilled Tomatoes

Servings: 2 lunch entrées (four blocks each)

Block Size:

2 Protein	2 whole eggs
2 Protein	6 ounces extra-firm tofu, diced fine
4 Protein and 4 Carbohydrate	2 cups plain low-fat yogurt
1 Carbohydrate	4 teaspoons cornstarch
3 Carbohydrate	3¾ cups tomato, diced
8 Fat	24 black olives, sliced

2 teaspoons mustard
2 garlic cloves, minced
⅛ teaspoon white wine
2 tablespoons dried dill
Lemon herb seasoning
Salt and pepper to taste

Method:
In nonstick saucepan, add yogurt, mustard, eggs, garlic, wine, and dill. Cook for 5–10 minutes until mixture is hot, then add cornstarch. (Mix cornstarch with a little water, then add to saucepan.) Stirring constantly, heat until a thick sauce forms, then add tomato, black olives, and tofu. Continue simmering for 2–3 minutes. Do not over-cook, as tomato and tofu will start to break down. Place an equal amount of the creamy dilled tomatoes on two lunch plates, then sprinkle with lemon herb seasoning and serve.

Turkey Burger Casserole

Servings: 2 lunch entrées (four blocks each)

Block Size:

6 Protein	9 ounces ground turkey
2 Protein	2 whole eggs
2 Carbohydrate	2 cups onion, minced
⅔ Carbohydrate	2 cups mushrooms, minced
2 Carbohydrate	½ cup cooked chickpeas
2 Carbohydrate	½ cup cooked kidney beans
⅔ Carbohydrate	1½ cups green bell pepper, diced
⅔ Carbohydrate	1½ cups red bell pepper, diced
8 Fat	2⅔ teaspoons olive oil

4 garlic cloves, minced, divided
⅛ teaspoon dried basil
⅛ teaspoon dried marjoram
⅛ teaspoon black pepper
⅛ teaspoon chili powder
⅛ teaspoon dried oregano
⅛ teaspoon paprika
⅛ teaspoon cayenne pepper
Salt to taste

Method:

In medium bowl, mix together ground turkey, eggs, onion, mushrooms, garlic, basil, marjoram, and black pepper. Form into two oblong loaf-shaped patties and place in baking pan. The loaf-shaped patties may be very sticky and loose; however, the egg will help the patties firm up as they bake. Bake in a preheated 375-degree oven for 30–35 minutes. While the turkey patties are cooking, add oil to nonstick sauté pan and cook chickpeas, kidney beans, peppers, chili powder, oregano, paprika, and cayenne pepper until hot. Using a large spatula, remove turkey patties from baking pan and place one on each lunch plate. Place an equal amount of vegetables on each plate and serve.

Malaysian Chicken Ball Soup

Servings: 2 lunch entrées (four blocks each)

Block Size:

8 Protein	12 ounces ground chicken
½ Carbohydrate	½ cup onion, diced fine
1½ Carbohydrate	1½ cups onion, sliced into half rings
2 Carbohydrate	2 cups leeks, halved and sliced
2 Carbohydrate	6 cups mushrooms, sliced
2 Carbohydrate	8 teaspoons cornstarch
8 Fat	2⅔ teaspoons olive oil
	12 drops hot sauce
	1 teaspoon parsley
	2 tablespoons grated ginger root*
	4 cups chicken stock
	Salt and pepper to taste

Method:
In a large bowl, combine chicken, diced onion, hot sauce, parsley, and ginger root. Form mixture into small half-inch meatballs. Place meatballs in baking dish brushed with oil and bake in a preheated 375-degree oven for 15 minutes. While the meatballs are cooking, put chicken stock in saucepan and bring to a boil. Add onion, leeks, and mushrooms. Cook vegetables in chicken stock until they are tender, then mix cornstarch with a little water and add to saucepan. Simmer for 3–5 minutes, stirring constantly until thickened. Remove meatballs from oven and add to saucepan. Place an equal amount of soup and meatballs in two soup bowls and serve immediately.

Note: When a recipe calls for fresh ginger root (available in most supermarkets or in Asian grocery stores), it is not advisable to substitute ground ginger. The flavors are very different.

Mexican Burger

Servings: 2 lunch entrées (four blocks each)

Block Size:

8 Protein	12 ounces ground beef
2 Carbohydrate	1 cup salsa
2 Carbohydrate	½ cup cooked kidney beans
2 Carbohydrate	2½ cups green bell pepper, diced
2 Carbohydrate	1 cup tomato puree
8 Fat	2⅔ teaspoons olive oil
	⅛ teaspoon chili powder or to taste
	⅛ teaspoon hot sauce or to taste
	Salt and pepper to taste

Method:

In a medium bowl, mix together the ground beef and salsa. Form into 2 oblong patties and place under broiler. Cook until browned. While the patties are cooking, add oil to nonstick sauté pan and cook kidney beans and peppers until hot, then add chili powder, hot sauce, and tomato puree. Simmer for 5 minutes, stirring constantly. Remove patties from broiler and place a patty on each lunch plate. Place an equal amount of vegetables on each plate and serve.

Hamburger Pie

Servings: 2 lunch entrées (four blocks each)

Block Size:

8 Protein	12 ounces ground beef
1 Carbohydrate	1 cup cooked turnips, mashed
1 Carbohydrate	1 cup onion, diced
2 Carbohydrate	2 cups mushrooms, diced fine, plus 4 cups mushrooms, diced fine

2 Carbohydrate	2 cups green beans, sliced
1 Carbohydrate	1¼ cups tomato, chopped
1 Carbohydrate	4 teaspoons cornstarch
8 Fat	2⅔ teaspoons olive oil
	3 teaspoons Worcestershire sauce
	¼ teaspoon dried marjoram
	¼ teaspoon dried oregano
	⅛ teaspoon dried thyme
	⅛ teaspoon dried sage
	¼ teaspoon black pepper
	2 garlic cloves, minced
	½ cup beef stock
	Salt to taste

Method:

In saucepan, place turnips in enough water to cover. Cook until tender. Drain water from saucepan, and using a masher, mash turnips to a smooth consistency. In nonstick sauté pan, add ⅔ teaspoon oil, ground beef, Worcestershire sauce, onion, and 2 cups diced fine mushrooms. Cook until ground beef is browned. In another nonstick sauté pan, place remaining oil, 4 cups diced fine mushrooms, green beans, tomato, and spices. Cook until vegetables are tender. While the vegetables are cooking, in a small mixing bowl combine garlic, beef stock, and cornstarch. When the vegetables are cooked, add contents of mixing bowl to vegetables and continue heating until a sauce forms. Evenly coat vegetables with sauce. Layer two small baking dishes with beef mixture, then the vegetables and sauce mixture, and lastly the mashed turnips. Bake in preheated 350-degree oven for 10–15 minutes until the mashed turnips top has browned. Place on two lunch plates and serve immediately.

Louisiana-Style Shrimp

Servings: 2 lunch entrées (four blocks each)

Block Size:

7 Protein	10½ ounces cooked shrimp (20 count)
1 Protein and 1 Carbohydrate	1 cup 1 percent milk
1½ Carbohydrate	3 cups green bell pepper, half rings
1½ Carbohydrate	3 cups red bell pepper, half rings
2 Carbohydrate	2 cups onion, sliced
1 Carbohydrate	2 cups celery
1 Carbohydrate	½ cup tomato puree
1 Carbohydrate	4 teaspoons cornstarch
8 Fat	2⅔ teaspoons olive oil
	2 tablespoons cider vinegar
	1 cup water
	⅛ teaspoon hot sauce (or to taste)
	⅛ teaspoon celery salt
	Black pepper to taste

Method:

In nonstick sauté pan add oil, bell pepper half rings, onion, celery, and vinegar. Cook until vegetables are tender, then add shrimp, milk, water, tomato puree, hot sauce, seasonings, and cornstarch. (Mix cornstarch with a little water before adding it to the sauté pan, so that the cornstarch is dissolved.) Bring mixture slowly to a boil, then simmer for 5–10 minutes. Equally divide between two soup bowls and serve.

Stuffed Curry Peppers

Servings: 2 lunch entrées (four blocks each)

Block Size:

2 Protein	2 whole eggs
6 Protein	18 ounces extra-firm tofu
2 Carbohydrate	2 cups onion, diced fine
1 Carbohydrate	3 cups mushrooms, diced fine
2 Carbohydrate	½ cup cooked kidney beans, chopped
1 Carbohydrate	2¼ cups red bell pepper, diced fine
2 Carbohydrate	4 green peppers
8 Fat	2⅔ teaspoons olive oil

4 garlic cloves, minced
2 teaspoons hot curry powder
½ teaspoon dry mustard
⅛ teaspoon celery salt
⅛ teaspoon cinnamon
⅛ teaspoon black pepper
¼ teaspoon turmeric
⅛ teaspoon chili powder
⅛ teaspoon hot sauce (or to taste)
Salt to taste

Method:
In nonstick sauté pan, add oil, onion, garlic, mushrooms, kidney beans, and red bell pepper. Cook until vegetables are tender, then remove from heat and cool. In a mixing bowl, place cooked vegetable mixture, eggs, tofu, spices, and hot sauce. Mix well until all ingredients have been combined. Cut the stem top off the green peppers and remove the seeds inside, also if necessary cut a little off the bottom of the green pepper to allow the green pepper to stand still without moving. Stuff green peppers with tofu vegetable mixture and place in baking dish. If there is any vegetable mixture left over place around green peppers. Tightly seal baking dish with

aluminum foil and bake in a preheated oven at 400 degrees for 1 hour. Remove baking dish from oven and place two stuffed peppers on each lunch plate. Serve immediately.

Thai Green Fish Curry

Servings: 2 lunch entrées (four blocks each)

Block Size:

6 Protein	9 ounces fresh fish fillets, cut in slivers
2 Protein and 2 Carbohydrate	1 cup plain low-fat yogurt
2 Carbohydrate	2 cups snow peas, whole
2 Carbohydrate	2 cups onion, chopped
1 Carbohydrate	1½ cups hot peppers, in rings
1 Carbohydrate	4 teaspoons cornstarch
8 Fat	2⅔ teaspoons olive oil

4 garlic cloves, minced
4 teaspoons vinegar
1½ cups water
1 teaspoon turmeric
4 teaspoons hot curry powder
Salt and pepper to taste

Method:
In nonstick sauté pan add oil, snow peas, onion, garlic, hot peppers, and vinegar. Cook until vegetables are tender, then add fish, yogurt, water, and spices. Cover sauté pan and poach fish in vegetable liquid until cooked though. When the fish is cooked, mix the cornstarch with a little water and add to sauté pan. Bring mixture to a boil, then simmer for an additional 5–10 minutes. Equally divide between two soup bowls and serve.

Vegetarian Franks and Beans

Servings: 2 lunch entrées (four blocks each)

Block Size:

8 Protein	8 soy hot dogs
6 Carbohydrate	1½ cups cooked black beans
1 Carbohydrate	1 cup onion, chopped fine
1 Carbohydrate	½ cup tomato puree
8 Fat	2⅔ teaspoons olive oil
	2 garlic cloves, minced
	1 teaspoon dry mustard
	½ cup water

Method:
In nonstick sauté pan, add oil, black beans, and onion. Cook black beans and onion until hot, then add garlic, mustard, tomato puree, water, and soy hot dogs. Cover sauté pan and simmer for 5–10 minutes until soy hot dogs are hot, occasionally stirring. Equally divide the beans and franks between two lunch plates. Place four soy hot dogs and an equal amount of beans on each plate and serve immediately.

Sweet and Sour Pork and Cabbage

Servings: 2 lunch entrées (four blocks each)

Block Size:

8 Protein	8 ounces pork loin, in half-inch cubes
2 Carbohydrate	6 cups cabbage, shredded
4 Carbohydrate	1 cup cooked chickpeas, chopped
2 Carbohydrate	6 cups mushrooms, sliced
8 Fat	2⅔ teaspoons olive oil
	10 tablespoons cider vinegar
	½ cup water
	Salt and pepper to taste

Method:
Sprinkle pork with salt and pepper, then place in nonstick sauté pan with ⅓ teaspoon oil. Cook until pork is browned. When the pork is cooked, remove it from pan and set aside. Add cabbage, chickpeas, mushrooms, vinegar, and 2 teaspoons oil to sauté pan and cook vegetable mixture for about 10–15 minutes, until vegetables are almost tender. Add water and cooked pork to vegetables in sauté pan. Cover sauté pan and braise mixture for 5–10 minutes, stirring occasionally. Divide between two lunch plates and serve.

Beef Chop Suey

Servings: 2 lunch entrées (four blocks each)

Block Size:

8 Protein	8 ounces beef eye of round, one-eighth-inch slices

1 Carbohydrate	3 cups cabbage, shredded
1 Carbohydrate	2 cups celery, willow leaf cut*
½ Carbohydrate	1½ cups mushrooms, sliced
½ Carbohydrate	1½ cups bean sprouts
1 Carbohydrate	½ cup water chestnuts
½ Carbohydrate	½ cup onion, chopped

8 Fat	2⅔ teaspoons olive oil

2 tablespoons cider vinegar
1 tablespoon low-sodium soy sauce
½ cup beef stock
2 teaspoons Worcestershire sauce

Method:
In nonstick sauté pan, place ⅔ teaspoon oil and beef. Cook beef until browned and done. While the beef is cooking, in another nonstick sauté pan place 2 teaspoons oil, cabbage, celery, mushrooms, bean sprouts, water chestnuts, vinegar, and onion. Cook until entire mixture is hot, then add soy sauce, beef stock, beef, and Worcestershire sauce. Cover sauté pan and cook for 5–10 minutes, stirring occasionally to blend flavors. Place an equal amount on two lunch plates and serve.

*Note: Willow leaf cut means that the celery is cut at approximately a 45-degree angle. Also, there is no need to add any salt to this dish, because celery is naturally high in sodium.

Vegetarian Hot Dog Casserole

Servings: 2 lunch entrées (four blocks each)

Block Size:

8 Protein	8 soy hot dogs, sliced
2 Carbohydrate	6 cups cabbage, shredded
2 Carbohydrate	6 cups mushrooms, sliced
2 Carbohydrate	½ cup cooked chickpeas, chopped
2 Carbohydrate	½ cup carrots, willow leaf cut*
8 Fat	2⅔ teaspoons olive oil

2 garlic cloves, minced
6 tablespoons cider vinegar
2 teaspoons fresh mint, chopped
½ cup water

Method:
In nonstick sauté pan, add oil, cabbage, mushrooms, chickpeas, and carrots. Cook vegetable mixture until hot, then add garlic, vinegar, mint, water, and soy hot dogs. Cover sauté pan and simmer for 5–10 minutes until soy hot dogs are hot, occasionally stirring. Equally divide the cooked vegetables and franks between two lunch plates. Place four soy hot dogs and an equal amount of vegetables on each plate and serve immediately.

Note: Willow leaf cut means that the carrots are cut at approximately a 45-degree angle.

Veal Stew

Servings: 2 lunch entrées (four blocks each)

Block Size:

8 Protein	8 ounces veal, one-inch cubes
1 Carbohydrate	3 cups mushroom caps
2 Carbohydrate	2 cups pearl onion
2 Carbohydrate	2 cups cherry tomato
2 Carbohydrate	2 cups turnips, cut Parisienne style*
1 Carbohydrate	4 teaspoons cornstarch
8 Fat	2⅔ teaspoons olive oil

2 garlic cloves, minced
1 cup beef stock
6 whole peppercorns
¼ teaspoon dried oregano
2 teaspoons fresh basil, chopped
Salt and pepper to taste

Method:
Coat bottom of medium-sized casserole dish with oil. Place all ingredients (veal, vegetables, and spices) in casserole dish, except basil and cornstarch. Tightly cover casserole dish with aluminum foil and place in preheated oven at 400 degrees for 20 minutes. Mix the cornstarch and basil together with a little water to form a paste. After 20 minutes, remove casserole dish from oven and stir in cornstarch-basil paste. Continue stirring meat and vegetables until they have been coated. Re-cover and cook an additional 5–10 minutes. Place equal amount of veal pieces on two lunch plates and top with vegetables and sauce.

Note: Use a small melon ball cutter on turnips to form small balls.

Tuna Fruit Salad

Servings: 2 lunch entrées (four blocks each)

Block Size:

7 Protein	7 ounces chunk light tuna, drained*
1 Protein and 1 Carbohydrate	½ cup plain low-fat yogurt
2 Carbohydrate	1 cup blueberries
2 Carbohydrate	2 cups strawberries, sliced
2 Carbohydrate	⅔ cup mandarin orange sections
1 Carbohydrate	6 cups romaine lettuce, chopped
8 Fat	8 teaspoons slivered almonds
	½ teaspoon parsley flakes
	½ teaspoon dried dill
	⅛ teaspoon onion powder
	⅛ teaspoon nutmeg
	⅛ teaspoon paprika
	Salt and pepper to taste

Method:

In a small mixing bowl, combine tuna (without liquid), yogurt, parsley, dill, onion powder, and nutmeg to form a tuna salad. In another mixing bowl, combine blueberries, strawberries, and orange sections to form a fruit salad. When the tuna salad and fruit salad are made, take two lunch plates and arrange a bed of lettuce on each plate. In the center of the plate on the bed of lettuce place a mound of tuna salad. Place the fruit salad around the tuna salad and sprinkle with paprika and slivered almonds. Chill and serve.

Note: Use tuna packed in water only.

Chicken Salad Mexicana

Servings: 2 lunch entrées (four blocks each)

Block Size:

8 Protein	8 ounces chicken tenderloins, diced (or skinless chicken breast)
1 Carbohydrate	2 cups celery, diced
2 Carbohydrate	½ cup cooked chickpeas, chopped
2 Carbohydrate	½ cup cooked kidney beans, chopped
2 Carbohydrate	1 cup salsa*
1 Carbohydrate	6 cups romaine lettuce
8 Fat	2⅔ teaspoons olive oil

⅛ teaspoon chili powder
2 garlic cloves, minced
⅛ teaspoon Worcestershire sauce
Onion powder
Salt and pepper to taste

Method:
In nonstick sauté pan, add oil, diced chicken, celery, chili powder, garlic, and Worcestershire sauce. Cook until chicken is browned, then add chickpeas, kidney beans, and salsa. Simmer for 10–15 minutes until heated through and beans have softened. The kidney beans should have a soft consistency like refried beans. While the chicken and vegetables are cooking, take two lunch plates and arrange a bed of lettuce on both plates. Remove sauté pan from stove and let chicken and vegetable mixture cool for 2–3 minutes. Spoon chicken and vegetable mixture into the center of both plates on each bed of lettuce. Sprinkle with onion powder and serve.

Note: Salsa comes with different levels of heat. Choose one that best fits your family's tastes.

Thousand Island Salad

Servings: 2 lunch entrées (four blocks each)

Block Size:

2 Protein	2 whole hard-boiled eggs, chopped
2 Protein	2 ounces skim milk mozzarella cheese, shredded
1 Protein	1½ ounces deli-style turkey breast, diced
1 Protein	1½ ounces deli-style ham, diced
2 Protein and 2 Carbohydrate	1 cup plain low-fat yogurt
2 Carbohydrate	8 teaspoons sweet pickle relish
1 Carbohydrate	1 head iceberg lettuce
1 Carbohydrate	1 cup cherry tomato, halved
½ Carbohydrate	½ cup onion, diced fine
½ Carbohydrate	1 cup radishes, sliced
1 Carbohydrate	½ cup tomato puree
8 Fat	24 green olives, chopped
	⅛ teaspoon chili powder
	⅛ teaspoon Worcestershire sauce
	Salt and pepper to taste

Method:

In a small mixing bowl, add yogurt, hard-boiled eggs, tomato puree, relish, olives, chili powder, and Worcestershire sauce. Blend together with a wire whip to create the dressing for the salad. When the dressing has been made, take two large oval plates and arrange a bed of lettuce on each plate. On each bed of lettuce, place an equal amount of tomato, onion, radishes, cheese, turkey, and ham. Equally divide the dressing and pour over salad ingredients on both plates. Sprinkle with salt and pepper and serve immediately.

Hot Spinach Salad

Servings: 2 lunch entrées (four blocks each)

Block Size:

8 Protein	12 ounces lean ground pork
1 Carbohydrate	1 cup onion, diced fine
1 Carbohydrate	4 teaspoons cornstarch
2 Carbohydrate	8 cups fresh spinach, stems removed and chopped*
4 Carbohydrate	1 cup cooked chickpeas, diced fine
8 Fat	2⅔ teaspoons olive oil

8 tablespoons cider vinegar
2 garlic cloves, minced
1 cup beef stock
½ teaspoon dry mustard
2 tablespoons red bell pepper, diced fine
Salt and pepper to taste

Method:
In nonstick sauté pan, add oil, pork, onion, vinegar, and garlic. Cook until pork is browned, stirring the pork as it cooks to break the pork up. When the pork has browned, add beef stock, mustard, and cornstarch. (Blend cornstarch and mustard with a little water to dissolve them before adding to sauté pan.) Bring pork mixture to a boil, stirring constantly until thickened and it develops into the hot spinach dressing. On two lunch plates, place 4 cups of cleaned raw spinach per plate. Equally divide hot spinach dressing (pork mixture) between both serving plates by spooning over spinach. Sprinkle each plate with chopped chickpeas and red bell pepper and serve.

Note: Fresh spinach needs to be cleaned very well, because of sand, so be sure to soak spinach in water to remove any sand or dirt before using.

Shrimp with Tri-Bean Salad

Servings: 2 lunch entrées (four blocks each)

Block Size:

8 Protein	12 ounces shrimp
2 Carbohydrate	½ cup cooked kidney beans
2 Carbohydrate	½ cup cooked chickpeas
2 Carbohydrate	2 cups green beans, diagonal cut
1 Carbohydrate	1 cup onion, chopped
1 Carbohydrate	6 cups romaine lettuce, diced
8 Fat	2⅔ teaspoons olive oil

2 tablespoons cider vinegar
2 tablespoons dried chives
⅛ teaspoon dried basil
⅛ teaspoon black pepper
⅛ teaspoon white wine
4 bay leaves
⅛ teaspoon parsley
Salt to taste

Method:

In a small mixing bowl, combine, oil, vinegar, chives, basil, black pepper, kidney beans, chickpeas, green beans, and onion to form a Tri-Bean Salad. Place mixing bowl in refrigerator to allow vegetables to marinate. In saucepan, poach shrimp in boiling water with wine and bay leaves until cooked. Remove shrimp from saucepan and cool. Arrange a bed of lettuce on two large plates. In the center of the plates on the lettuce place a mound of salad. Place the shrimp around the salad and sprinkle with parsley. Chill and serve.

Herbed Cottage Cheese and Asparagus Salad with Fruit

Servings: 2 lunch entrées (four blocks each)

Block Size:

8 Protein	2 cups low-fat cottage cheese
2 Carbohydrate	2 cups cooked asparagus, cut in one-inch pieces
2 Carbohydrate	2 peaches, sliced
2 Carbohydrate	⅔ cup mandarin orange sections
1 Carbohydrate	1 cup strawberries
1 Carbohydrate	6 cups romaine lettuce
8 Fat	2⅔ teaspoons olive oil
	⅛ teaspoon dried oregano
	2 teaspoons fresh basil, diced fine
	⅛ teaspoon black pepper
	⅛ teaspoon parsley
	Salt to taste

Method:

In a mixing bowl, combine cottage cheese, asparagus, oil, oregano, basil, and black pepper. In another mixing bowl, combine peaches, orange sections, and strawberries to form a fruit salad. When the herbed cottage cheese and fruit salad are made, take two lunch plates and arrange a bed of lettuce on each plate. In the center of the plate on the lettuce place a mound of herbed cottage cheese. Place the fruit salad around the herbed cottage cheese and sprinkle with parsley. Chill and serve.

Stuffed Tomato with Chicken Farce

Servings: 2 lunch entrées (four blocks each)

Block Size:

8 Protein	12 ounces ground chicken
2 Carbohydrate	4 tomatoes, crowned and cut in half
2 Carbohydrate	2 cups onion, diced fine
1 Carbohydrate	3 cups mushrooms, diced fine
1 Carbohydrate	½ cup carrots, diced fine
2 Carbohydrate	½ cup cooked chickpeas, chopped
8 Fat	2⅔ teaspoons olive oil
	Salt and pepper to taste
	4 teaspoons parsley
	2 garlic cloves, minced

Method:
Using a knife, cut tomatoes in half in a crown pattern. To crown a tomato, cut a zigzag line around the middle of the tomato with a sharp paring knife. When the two halves are separated, the top and bottom form bases that create the appearance of a crown. After the tomatoes have been cut, carefully cut out or scoop out the inside of the tomato to create a tomato shell. Sprinkle the insides of the tomato shells with salt and pepper. Dice tomato pulp into small chunks. In nonstick sauté pan add oil, onion, mushrooms, carrots, chickpeas, tomato pulp, parsley, garlic, and ground chicken. Cook until mixture is tender and chicken is browned (about 10 minutes). (This mixture is known as a duxell-farce. A *duxell-farce* is finely cooked vegetables and meat used to stuff another item.) When the duxell-farce is cooked, set aside to cool. Stuff crowned tomatoes with duxell-farce, then place in a baking dish. Tightly cover baking dish with aluminum foil and place in preheated oven at 350 degrees for 10–15 minutes to soften the tomatoes. Remove baking dish from oven and place four stuffed tomatoes on both lunch plates. Sprinkle with salt and pepper and serve immediately.

Barbecue Beef with Onions

Servings: 2 lunch entrées (four blocks each)

Block Size:

8 Protein	8 ounces beef eye of round, one-eighth-inch slices
4 Carbohydrate	2 cups tomato puree
4 Carbohydrate	4 cups onion, in half rings
8 Fat	2⅔ teaspoons olive oil

1 teaspoon Worcestershire sauce
1 teaspoon cider vinegar
½ teaspoon chili powder
⅛ teaspoon dried oregano
¼ teaspoon minced garlic
2 tablespoons beef stock
2 tablespoons white wine vinegar

Method:
In nonstick sauté pan, add ⅔ teaspoon oil and beef. Cook beef until browned. When the beef has browned, add tomato puree, Worcestershire sauce, cider vinegar, chili powder, oregano, and garlic. Cover and simmer for 5 minutes until a sauce forms. While the beef is simmering, in another nonstick sauté pan add remaining oil and onion. Cook onion until tender, then add the onion, beef stock, and white wine vinegar to beef. Cover sauté pan and cook 10 minutes, stirring occasionally to blend flavors. Place an equal amount on two lunch plates or in soup bowls and serve.

Creole Shrimp

Servings: 2 lunch entrées (four blocks each)

Block Size:

8 Protein	12 ounces cooked shrimp
1 Carbohydrate	1 cup onion, quarter-inch dice
1 Carbohydrate	2¼ cups green bell pepper, quarter-inch dice
1 Carbohydrate	2½ cups celery, quarter-inch dice
3 Carbohydrate	1½ cups tomato puree
2 Carbohydrate	2 peaches
8 Fat	2⅔ teaspoons olive oil

2 garlic cloves, minced
Hot sauce to taste
½ cup water
⅛ teaspoon celery salt
½ teaspoon dried thyme, crushed
⅛ teaspoon black pepper

Method:

In nonstick sauté pan, add oil, onion, pepper, celery, garlic, and hot sauce. Cook until vegetables are tender, then add shrimp, tomato puree, water, celery salt, thyme, and black pepper. Bring mixture to a boil, then simmer for 5–10 minutes. Equally divide Creole Shrimp between two lunch plates and serve. Serve peaches on the side as a dessert.

Herbed Pork and Bean Stew

Servings: 2 lunch entrées (four blocks each)

Block Size:

8 Protein	12 ounces ground pork
4 Carbohydrate	1 cup cooked kidney beans
2 Carbohydrate	2 cups green beans, diagonal cut
1 Carbohydrate	1 cup onion, chopped
1 Carbohydrate	4 teaspoons cornstarch
8 Fat	2⅔ teaspoons olive oil

4 garlic cloves, minced
2 teaspoons cider vinegar
2 teaspoons Worcestershire sauce
1 cup chicken stock
⅛ teaspoon dried basil
½ teaspoon dried marjoram

Method:

In nonstick saucepan, cook kidney beans, green beans, garlic, and onion in 2 teaspoons oil until tender, then add vinegar, Worcestershire sauce, chicken stock, spices, and cornstarch. (Mix cornstarch with a little water to dissolve it before adding to sauté pan.) Continue cooking under medium heat until entire mixture is hot, stirring constantly. While the vegetables are cooking, in another nonstick sauté pan add remaining oil and stir-fry pork until cooked. When the pork is cooked, add it to the vegetables and simmer for an additional 5 minutes. Place an equal amount in two soup bowls and serve.

Fruity Chicken Salad

Servings: 2 lunch entrées (four blocks each)

Block Size:

8 Protein	8 ounces chicken tenderloins, diced (or skinless chicken breast)

4 Carbohydrate	1 cantaloupe
1 Carbohydrate	½ cup blueberries
1 Carbohydrate	¾ cup maraschino cherries
1 Carbohydrate	1 kiwi fruit, peeled and diced
1 Carbohydrate	1 cup raspberries

8 Fat	2⅔ teaspoons olive oil

Method:

In nonstick sauté pan, add oil and chicken. Cook chicken until browned. Remove chicken from sauté pan and let cool. Using a knife, cut cantaloupe in half in a crown pattern. To crown a cantaloupe, cut a zigzag line around the middle of the cantaloupe with a sharp paring knife. When the two halves are separated, the top and bottom form bases that create the appearance of a crown. After the cantaloupe has been cut, carefully cut out or scoop out the inside of the cantaloupe using a melon baller. Create a cavity inside the melon, leaving about a half inch of the melon on the rind. In a small mixing bowl, combine cantaloupe balls, blueberries, cherries, diced kiwi fruit, raspberries, and diced chicken to make a chicken-fruit salad. Divide chicken-fruit salad equally and fill the two cantaloupe halves, place on two lunch plates, and serve.

Beef and Lentil Stew

Servings: 2 lunch entrées (four blocks each)

Block Size:

8 Protein	8 ounces beef eye of round, diced in one-eighth-inch squares
1 Carbohydrate	½ cup tomato puree
1 Carbohydrate	½ cup carrots, diced fine
1 Carbohydrate	1 cup onion, diced fine
1 Carbohydrate	2½ cups celery, diced fine
4 Carbohydrates	½ cup dry lentils
8 Fat	2⅔ teaspoons olive oil

4 peppercorns, crushed
4 garlic cloves, minced
⅛ teaspoon dried marjoram
⅛ teaspoon dried basil
1 teaspoon parsley
4 cups beef stock

Method:
Combine all ingredients in large saucepan. Bring to a boil, then simmer for 35–40 minutes. Divide between two soup dishes and serve.

Spanish Chicken and Lentil Soup

Servings: 2 lunch entrées (four blocks each)

Block Size:

6 Protein	6 ounces chicken tenderloins, diced fine (or skinless chicken breast)
2 Protein and 2 Carbohydrate	1 cup plain low-fat yogurt
4 Carbohydrate	1 cup cooked lentils
1 Carbohydrate	½ cup tomato puree
½ Carbohydrate	½ cup onion, chopped fine
½ Carbohydrate	3 cups fresh spinach, shredded
8 Fat	2⅔ teaspoons olive oil
	⅛ teaspoon dried parsley
	⅛ teaspoon dried thyme
	⅛ teaspoon dried basil
	⅛ teaspoon dried rosemary
	1 cup chicken stock

Method:

In a large nonstick sauté pan, add ⅔ teaspoon oil and chicken. Cook chicken over medium heat until browned, then add cooked lentils, tomato puree, onion, spinach, spices, and chicken stock. Continue cooking until entire mixture is hot and has come to a boil. Simmer for 5 minutes, remove from heat, and stir in yogurt. Place an equal amount in two soup bowls and serve.

Beef Ratatouille

Servings: 2 lunch entrées (four blocks each)

Block Size:

8 Protein	12 ounces lean ground beef
2 Carbohydrate	3 cups zucchini, quartered
2 Carbohydrate	2 cups onion, half-ring slices
2 Carbohydrate	2½ cups tomato, half slices
2 Carbohydrate	4½ cups red bell pepper, diced
8 Fat	2⅔ teaspoons olive oil

6 garlic cloves, minced
2 tablespoons dried basil
⅛ teaspoon dried oregano
½ cup beef stock

Method:
In nonstick sauté pan, place ⅔ teaspoon oil and beef. Cook beef until browned and done. In another sauté pan, place 2 teaspoons oil, zucchini, onion, tomato, bell pepper, garlic, basil, and oregano. Cook until entire mixture is hot, then add beef stock and cooked beef. Cover sauté pan and cook for 5–10 minutes, stirring occasionally to blend flavors. Place an equal amount on two lunch plates and serve.

Cinnamon-Chicken Meatballs with Fruit Sauce

Servings: 2 lunch entrées (four blocks each)

Block Size:

8 Protein	12 ounces ground chicken
1 Carbohydrate	1 cup onion, diced fine
1 Carbohydrate	2 cups celery, diced fine, divided
2 Carbohydrate	½ cup kidney beans, chopped fine
1 Carbohydrate	4 teaspoons cornstarch
2 Carbohydrate	1 cup fruit cocktail
1 Carbohydrate	¾ cup maraschino cherries, halved
8 Fat	2⅔ teaspoons olive oil
	⅛ teaspoon black pepper
	1 teaspoon cinnamon plus ⅛ teaspoon
	1½ cups chicken stock
	½ teaspoon orange extract

Method:

In a large bowl, combine ground chicken, onion, 1 cup celery, finely chopped kidney beans, olive oil, black pepper, and 1 teaspoon cinnamon. Form mixture into 32 one-inch meatballs. Place meatballs in baking dish and bake in a preheated 375-degree oven for 15 minutes. While the meatballs are cooking, in a small saucepan combine fruit cocktail, cherries, 1 cup celery, chicken stock, ⅛ teaspoon cinnamon, orange extract, and cornstarch. (Mix cornstarch with chicken stock so that it can dissolve before adding to saucepan.) Simmer lightly until sauce forms, stirring constantly. Remove meatballs from oven and place meatballs in sauce, gently spooning the sauce over the meatballs. Place an equal amount of meatballs on two lunch plates with sauce and serve.

Greek Chicken Stew

Servings: 2 lunch entrées (four blocks each)

Block Size:

8 Protein	8 ounces chicken tenderloins, diced fine (or skinless chicken breast)
2 Carbohydrate	2 cups onion, sliced thin
2 Carbohydrate	1 cup tomato puree
2 Carbohydrate	2 cups fresh green beans, chopped
1 Carbohydrate	½ cup carrots, chopped
1 Carbohydrate	1 cup turnips, one-eighth-inch cubes
8 Fat	24 pitted black olives, sliced (or similar type)

2 garlic cloves, minced
2 cups chicken stock*
⅛ teaspoon red wine
⅛ teaspoon celery salt
⅛ teaspoon pepper
½ teaspoon cinnamon

Method:
Combine all ingredients except olives in a large saucepan. Bring to a boil, then simmer for 30–35 minutes, stirring occasionally, until all vegetables are tender. Add olives and divide between two soup dishes and serve.

*Note: If more chicken stock is needed or a more liquid stew is desired, add additional stock as necessary.

Rich and Hearty Minestrone Soup

Servings: 2 lunch entrées (four blocks each)

Block Size:

8 Protein	8 ounces beef eye of round, diced in one-eighth-inch squares
1 Carbohydrate	2½ cups celery, diced fine
1 Carbohydrate	1 cup onion, diced fine
1 Carbohydrate	3 cups cabbage, diced fine
1 Carbohydrate	½ cup tomato puree
1 Carbohydrate	⅛ cup cooked black beans
1 Carbohydrate	⅛ cup cooked chickpeas
1 Carbohydrate	¼ cup cooked elbow macaroni
8 Fat	2⅔ teaspoons olive oil
	2 garlic cloves, minced
	3 cups beef stock
	Salt and pepper to taste
	½ teaspoon dried basil

Method:

Combine all ingredients except macaroni in a large saucepan. Bring to a boil, then simmer for 30–35 minutes, stirring occasionally, until all vegetables are tender. While the soup is cooking, add macaroni to boiling water and cook. When macaroni is cooked, remove from water and cool until it is time to add the macaroni to the soup. Add macaroni and simmer for an additional 5 minutes. Divide between two soup dishes and serve.

Home-Style Beef-Vegetable Soup

Servings: 2 lunch entrées (four blocks each)

Block Size:

8 Protein	12 ounces lean ground beef
1 Carbohydrate	2½ cups celery, diced fine
2 Carbohydrate	1 cup carrots, diced fine
2 Carbohydrate	2 cups onion, diced fine
2 Carbohydrate	2½ cups tomato, chopped
1 Carbohydrate	½ cup tomato puree
8 Fat	2⅔ teaspoons olive oil

3 cups beef stock
Salt and pepper to taste
4 green peppercorns
2 garlic cloves, minced
⅛ teaspoon marjoram
⅛ teaspoon Worcestershire sauce
¼ teaspoon chives
1 teaspoon parsley
⅛ teaspoon oregano

Method:
Combine all ingredients in a large saucepan. Bring to a boil, then simmer for 35–40 minutes, stirring occasionally, until all vegetables are tender. Divide between two soup dishes and serve.

Variations:

Vegetable Soup Brunoise
Cut vegetable in a fine dice (one-eighth-inch cubes).

Vegetable Soup Paysanne
Means peasant style; the vegetables are cut in a coarse cut (one-quarter-inch cubes).

Thick Old-Fashioned Cabbage Soup

Servings: 2 lunch entrées (four blocks each)

Block Size:

8 Protein	8 soy hot dogs, sliced
1 Carbohydrate	2 cups celery, diced fine
2 Carbohydrate	1 cup carrots, diced fine
2 Carbohydrate	2 cups onion, diced fine
1 Carbohydrate	1¼ cups tomato, diced fine
1 Carbohydrate	3 cups cabbage, shredded
1 Carbohydrate	3 cups mushrooms, diced
8 Fat	2⅔ teaspoons olive oil

3 cups chicken stock
⅛ teaspoon caraway seeds
2 garlic cloves, minced
4 tablespoons cider vinegar
Salt and pepper to taste

Method:
Combine all ingredients in a large saucepan. Bring to a boil, then simmer for 35–40 minutes, stirring occasionally until all vegetables are tender. Divide between two soup dishes and serve.

Broiled Tuna Steak with Dill Sauce and Fruit

Servings: 2 lunch entrées (four blocks each)

Block Size:

7 Protein	12 ounces tuna steak
1 Protein and 1 Carbohydrate	½ cup plain low-fat yogurt
½ Carbohydrate	½ teaspoon sugar
½ Carbohydrate	2 teaspoons cornstarch
2 Carbohydrate	1 cup pineapple, cubed
1 Carbohydrate	½ cup blueberries
2 Carbohydrate	⅔ cup mandarin oranges
1 Carbohydrate	¾ cup maraschino cherries, halved
8 Fat	2⅔ teaspoons olive oil
	2 teaspoons dried dill
	2 teaspoons white wine
	Salt and pepper to taste

Method:
Coat the bottom of a baking dish with oil, then place two 6-ounce pieces of tuna in bottom of baking dish. Sprinkle with 1 teaspoon of the dill, then tightly seal baking dish and bake in preheated oven at 375 degrees for 25–30 minutes. While the tuna is baking, in saucepan combine yogurt, sugar, the rest of the dill, and wine to make a dill sauce. Add a little water to the cornstarch and then add it to dill sauce. Stirring constantly, heat sauce through but do not bring sauce to a boil. In a mixing bowl, combine pineapple, blueberries, orange sections, and cherries to make a fruit salad. Equally divide fruit salad between two lunch plates, then remove baking dish from oven. Using a large spatula, scoop out tuna and place one piece of tuna on each plate. Pour an equal amount of dill sauce over each piece of tuna and serve immediately.

Crabmeat Maryland

Servings: 2 lunch entrées (four blocks each)

Block Size:

8 Protein	12 ounces crabmeat, cut into half-inch pieces
1 Carbohydrate	2 cups celery, cut in matchstick-sized pieces (one-eighth-inch by one-eighth-inch by two inches)
1 Carbohydrate	1 cup onion, sliced in thin half rings
1 Carbohydrate	1 cup shallots, sliced in thin half rings
2 Carbohydrate	1 cup carrots, cut in matchstick-sized pieces (one-eighth inch by one-eighth inch by two inches)
1 Carbohydrate	1 cup tomato, diced fine
1 Carbohydrate	2¼ cups red bell pepper, in thin pieces
1 Carbohydrate	½ cup tomato puree
8 Fat	2⅔ teaspoons olive oil

4 garlic cloves, minced
1 cup chicken stock or fish stock
⅛ teaspoon red wine
⅛ teaspoon dried dill
⅛ teaspoon black pepper
⅛ teaspoon dried basil
Salt to taste

Method:

In nonstick sauté pan, add 2 teaspoons oil, celery, onion, shallots, carrots, diced tomato, garlic, and bell pepper. Cook until vegetables are tender, then add tomato puree, stock, red wine, and spices. Simmer for 10 minutes. While the vegetables are simmering, in another sauté pan add ⅔ teaspoon oil and crabmeat. Gently cook crabmeat until done, then add crabmeat to vegetable mixture and simmer an additional 5 minutes. Divide between two lunch plates and serve immediately.

Spicy Mexicali Beef

Servings: 2 lunch entrées (four blocks each)

Block Size:

8 Protein	10 ounces lean ground beef
1 Carbohydrate	¼ cup corn kernels
2 Carbohydrate	1 cup salsa
2 Carbohydrate	½ cup cooked white kidney beans, rinsed
2 Carbohydrate	½ cup cooked black beans, rinsed
1 Carbohydrate	1 cup tomato, seeded and diced fine
5 Fat	1⅔ teaspoons olive oil
3 Fat	9 black olives, diced

1 tablespoon chili powder
⅛ teaspoon celery salt
½ teaspoon onion powder
⅛ teaspoon cayenne pepper
½ teaspoon garlic, minced

Method:
In nonstick sauté pan, add ground beef and ⅔ teaspoon oil. When the beef has browned, add all remaining ingredients and cook for 10–15 minutes until hot. Place the mixture in two small bowls and serve.

Chicken Florida

Servings: 2 lunch entrées (four blocks each)

Block Size:

8 Protein	8 ounces chicken tenderloins, diced (or skinless chicken breast)
1 Carbohydrate	1 cup onion, chopped
1 Carbohydrate	1½ cups cooked spinach

1 Carbohydrate	2 cups red bell pepper, sliced and quartered
½ Carbohydrate	1½ cups mushrooms, sliced
½ Carbohydrate	1 cup broccoli florets
½ Carbohydrate	1½ cups cauliflower florets
1 Carbohydrate	1 cup asparagus spears, half-inch pieces
½ Carbohydrate	2 teaspoons cornstarch
2 Carbohydrate	½ cup cooked rotini pasta
8 Fat	2⅔ teaspoons olive oil, divided
	½ cup chicken stock
	¼ teaspoon black pepper
	¼ teaspoon chives, dried
	¼ teaspoon garlic, minced
	⅛ teaspoon tarragon, dried
	⅛ teaspoon thyme, dried
	⅛ teaspoon chili powder
	⅛ teaspoon celery salt

Method:

In a medium-sized nonstick sauté pan, add ⅔ teaspoon oil, onion, and spinach. Cook onion and spinach until spinach is wilted. In another nonstick sauté pan, add remaining oil, chicken, bell pepper, mushrooms, broccoli, cauliflower, and asparagus. Cook chicken and vegetables until done. In a small saucepan, combine chicken stock, spices, and cornstarch and stir until cornstarch has dissolved. Heat chicken stock until it has formed a sauce, then add rotini pasta to saucepan. On two lunch plates, place a mixture of onions and spinach, then place chicken mixture on top. Pour sauce over entire chicken-vegetable mixture and serve.

DINNER

Spinaci Chicken alla Italiana

(Spinach and Chicken Sautéed with Onion and Garlic)

Servings: 2 dinner entrées (four blocks each)

Block Size:

8 Protein	8 ounces skinless chicken breast, half-inch dice
4 Carbohydrate	1 pound fresh spinach, washed
3½ Carbohydrate	3½ cups onion, sliced thin
½ Carbohydrate	½ cup shallots, medium dice*
8 Fat	2⅔ teaspoons olive oil, divided

2 garlic cloves, minced (1 teaspoon)
⅛ teaspoon black pepper
½ teaspoon nutmeg
Fresh parsley sprigs
Salt to taste

Method:
In nonstick sauté pan, cook spinach, onion, garlic, and shallots in 2 teaspoons oil until tender. Just before the vegetables are finished cooking, add black pepper and nutmeg, remove pan from heat and set aside. In another nonstick sauté pan, cook diced chicken in ⅔ teaspoon olive oil until lightly browned, then add spinach mixture into diced chicken and heat through. Simmer entire mixture for 3–5 minutes. Place on two dinner plates and serve garnished with fresh parsley.

*Note: Shallots are available in most supermarkets and have a purple-white appearance. Shallots provide dishes with both an onion and a garlic flavor.

Hawaiian Sweet and Sour Chicken with Snow Peas

Servings: 2 dinner entrées (four blocks each)

Block Size:

8 Protein	8 ounces skinless chicken breast, half-inch dice
1 Carbohydrate	½ cup tomato puree
1 Carbohydrate	2 teaspoons sugar
2 Carbohydrate	1 cup pineapple, diced
1 Carbohydrate	¾ cup maraschino cherries, quartered
1 Carbohydrate	4 teaspoons cornstarch
2 Carbohydrate	2 cups snow peas
7 Fat	2⅓ teaspoons olive oil
1 Fat	1 teaspoon slivered almonds
	8 tablespoons vinegar
	4 tablespoons water
	2 tablespoons soy sauce
	1 cup chicken stock

Method:

In nonstick sauté pan, cook chicken in 2 teaspoons oil until done. While the chicken is cooking, in another nonstick sauté pan add vinegar, tomato puree, ⅓ teaspoon oil, water, soy sauce, sugar, pineapple, cherries, chicken stock, and cornstarch. (Mix cornstarch into chicken stock and stir well until cornstarch has dissolved before adding to saucepan.) While stirring continuously, heat pineapple and cherry mixture under medium heat until a thick sauce forms. Add chicken to pineapple and cherry mixture and simmer for 10 minutes for the flavors to blend. Taste sauce; if it has too strong a vinegar taste, continue simmering for a few more minutes. The flavor will develop into a sweet and sour sauce as it cooks. Place snow peas in saucepan with enough water to cover and cook until tender. Serve chicken mixture with peapods arranged on the sides of two dinner plates. Sprinkle almonds over snow peas and serve.

Chicken Fricassee with Garden Vegetables

Servings: 2 dinner entrées (four blocks each)

Block Size:

6 Protein	6 ounces skinless chicken breast, sliced in half-inch by two-inch strips
2 Protein and 2 Carbohydrate	1 cup plain low-fat yogurt
1 Carbohydrate	1 cup onion, sliced
1⅓ Carbohydrate	4 cups mushrooms, quartered
1 Carbohydrate	4 teaspoons cornstarch
1 Carbohydrate	1½ cups broccoli florets
⅔ Carbohydrate	2 cups mushrooms, sliced
8 Fat	8 teaspoons slivered almonds
	1½ cups chicken stock
	⅛ teaspoon lemon juice
	Salt and pepper to taste
	Red bell pepper strips for garnish (optional)

Method:

In saucepan, cook onions, quartered mushrooms, and chicken in chicken stock, until vegetables are tender and chicken is done. Remove saucepan from heat and slowly stir in lemon juice and yogurt, then add cornstarch. (Mix cornstarch with a little water and then add to saucepan.) Lightly simmer chicken mixture 4–5 minutes until mixture thickens. In another saucepan, place broccoli and enough water to cover. Cook broccoli until tender. Place Chicken Fricassee mixture on two serving plates along with an equal amount of cooked broccoli topped with sliced mushrooms and slivered almonds. Garnish with a red pepper strip and serve.

Clams à l'Ancienne

Servings: 2 dinner entrées (four blocks each)

Block Size:

4 Protein	6 ounces clams, chopped
2 Protein	2 whole eggs
2 Protein and 2 Carbohydrate	1 cup plain low-fat yogurt
2 Carbohydrate	4½ cups green bell pepper, chopped
1 Carbohydrate	3 cups mushrooms, diced
1 Carbohydrate	1 cup shallots, diced
2 Carbohydrate	2½ cups tomato, diced
1 Carbohydrate	4 teaspoons cornstarch
8 Fat	2⅔ teaspoons olive oil
	2 teaspoons hot sauce
	¼ teaspoon turmeric
	Salt and pepper to taste

Method:

In nonstick sauté pan, stir-fry all vegetables in hot oil until tender (2–3 minutes), then add clams and continue cooking until mixture is heated throughout. In a small mixing bowl, blend yogurt, eggs, hot sauce, seasonings, and cornstarch. (Mix cornstarch with a little water until it has dissolved before adding to mixing bowl.) After the ingredients in the mixing bowl have been mixed together, pour mixture into the sauté pan over clams and vegetable mixture. Stir well and cook an additional 3–5 minutes to heat through until eggs and yogurt are heated. Divide entrée onto two dinner plates and serve.

Indonesian–Javanese Chicken

Servings: 2 dinner entrées (four blocks each)

Block Size:

6 Protein	6 ounces chicken tenderloins, medium dice (or skinless chicken breast)
2 Protein and 2 Carbohydrate	2 cups 1 percent milk
1 Carbohydrate	1 cup onion, diced fine
⅓ Carbohydrate	½ cup jalapeño pepper, chopped fine
1 Carbohydrate	4 teaspoons cornstarch
2 Carbohydrate	6 cups cabbage, shredded
⅔ Carbohydrate	2 cups red bell pepper, sliced
8 Fat	2⅔ teaspoons olive oil
	6 garlic cloves, minced
	2 teaspoons ginger root, grated
	½ teaspoon turmeric
	1 teaspoon coriander
	½ teaspoon curry powder
	Salt and pepper to taste

Method:
In nonstick sauté pan, combine onion, jalapeño pepper, spices, milk, and chicken. Poach (lightly simmer) chicken in vegetable-milk mixture until cooked. Mix cornstarch with a little water, then add to sauté pan and simmer for 3–5 minutes. In a separate nonstick sauté pan, cook cabbage and red bell pepper in oil until tender. Divide cabbage and pepper between two dinner plates, then with a spoon equally divide chicken-vegetable mixture on the beds of cabbage and peppers. Serve immediately.

Chicken Chasseur

Servings: 2 dinner entrées (four blocks each)

Block Size:

8 Protein	Skinless breast pieces from 1-pound chicken, with the bone (approximately half the weight of this chicken breast is in bone) or 8 ounces skinless breast meat
4 Carbohydrate	5 cups tomato, diced
2 Carbohydrate	6 cups mushrooms, sliced
1 Carbohydrate	1 cup onion, sliced
1 Carbohydrate	4 teaspoons cornstarch
8 Fat	2⅔ teaspoons olive oil
	2 cups beef stock
	2 garlic cloves, minced
	⅛ teaspoon white wine
	Salt and pepper to taste

Method:
In a covered saucepan, poach (lightly simmer) chicken pieces in beef stock until cooked. In nonstick sauté pan, cook vegetables and garlic in oil over medium heat until tender, then add dash of wine. Mix cornstarch with a little water to dissolve it, then stir into beef stock with chicken to form a sauce. When the sauce has thickened, add vegetables and coat both chicken and vegetables with sauce. Simmer chicken and vegetables for 5–8 minutes. Place an equal amount of chicken pieces and vegetables on two dinner plates and serve.

Chicken with Rosemary

Servings: 2 dinner entrées (four blocks each)

Block Size:

6 Protein	6 ounces skinless chicken breast, sliced in half-inch by two-inch strips
2 Protein and 2 Carbohydrate	1 cup plain low-fat yogurt
1 Carbohydrate	4 teaspoons cornstarch
1 Carbohydrate	1½ cups broccoli florets
2 Carbohydrate	2½ cups tomato, sliced
2 Carbohydrate	1 pear, sliced
8 Fat	2⅔ teaspoons olive oil
	2 teaspoons dried rosemary
	1 cup chicken stock
	⅛ teaspoon paprika
	Salt and pepper to taste

Method:
In nonstick sauté pan, cook chicken in oil until lightly browned. When the chicken is cooked, add yogurt, paprika, and rosemary to sauté pan and simmer 3 minutes. Mix cornstarch with chicken stock and then add to sauté pan. Simmer until a sauce forms and the mixture thickens. While the chicken and sauce are simmering, place broccoli in saucepan with enough water to cover. Cook broccoli until tender. Prepare two dinner plates by placing a bed of tomato slices on each plate, topped with cooked broccoli. Place chicken and sauce beside broccoli and tomato slices on each plate. Garnish chicken with pear slices and serve.

Beef Stroganoff

Servings: 2 dinner entrées (four blocks each)

Block Size:

6 Protein	6 ounces beef eye of round, one-eighth-inch-thick slices
2 Protein and 2 Carbohydrate	1 cup plain low-fat yogurt
2 Carbohydrate	6 cups mushrooms, sliced
1 Carbohydrate	1 cup onion, diced fine
1 Carbohydrate	4 teaspoons cornstarch
2 Carbohydrate	2 cups green beans, French cut
8 Fat	2⅔ teaspoons olive oil
	⅛ teaspoon red wine
	⅛ teaspoon Worcestershire sauce
	½ cup beef stock
	2 tablespoons red bell pepper, diced fine
	Salt and pepper to taste

Method:

In nonstick sauté pan, cook mushrooms, onion, and beef in hot oil for 5–10 minutes. While the beef and vegetables are cooking in saucepan, combine wine, yogurt, Worcestershire sauce, beef stock, and cornstarch together to make a sauce. (Mix cornstarch with beef stock before adding to saucepan, so that the cornstarch can dissolve.) Simmer sauce, stirring occasionally until it has thickened and heated through; however, do not allow sauce to boil. When the sauce is hot, add the sauce to the mushrooms, onions, and beef, then simmer for 5 minutes. While the beef, vegetables, and sauce are simmering, in another saucepan, add green beans and red bell pepper with enough water to cover. Cook until tender. On two dinner plates, place an equal amount of Beef Stroganoff mixture and cooked green beans with red bell pepper. Serve immediately.

Vietnamese–Sweet Pork with Onions

Servings: 2 dinner entrées (four blocks each)

Block Size:

8 Protein	8 ounces pork, diced
8 Carbohydrate	8 cups onion, medium dice
8 Fat	2⅔ teaspoons olive oil
	½ cup beef stock
	4 tablespoons apple cider vinegar
	4 garlic cloves, chopped
	Salt and pepper to taste

Method:
In nonstick sauté pan, add diced oil, pork, and onion. Cook pork and onion over medium heat until both are browned. When onions have caramelized to a brown color, add beef stock, vinegar, and garlic. Bring mixture to a boil, then reduce heat and simmer for 30–45 minutes. Place an equal amount of the pork-onion mixture on two dinner plates and serve.

Swiss Steaks Jardiniere

Servings: 2 dinner entrées (four blocks each)

Block Size:

8 Protein	8 ounces beef eye of round, one-eighth-inch slices
2 Carbohydrate	1 cup tomato puree
1 Carbohydrate	2 cups celery, cut in matchstick-sized pieces (one-eighth inch by one-eighth inch by two inches)
2 Carbohydrate	2 cups onion, sliced in thin half rings

2 Carbohydrate

1 cup carrots, cut in matchstick-sized pieces (one-eighth inch by one-eighth inch by two inches)

1 Carbohydrate

2¼ cups red bell pepper

8 Fat

2⅔ teaspoons olive oil

1 cup beef stock
⅛ teaspoon red wine
4 garlic cloves, minced
⅛ teaspoon dried oregano
⅛ teaspoon black pepper
⅛ teaspoon dried basil
Salt to taste

Method:

In nonstick sauté pan, place ⅔ teaspoon of oil and beef. Cook beef until browned and done. After the beef has browned, add beef stock, tomato puree, and red wine. Continue cooking until a sauce forms and mixture is hot. In a second nonstick sauté pan, place 2 teaspoons oil and vegetables. Sprinkle vegetables with spices and cook until tender, stirring constantly. When the vegetables are cooked, add the beef mixture to the vegetables and simmer the entire mixture for 5 minutes. Place an equal amount of beef and vegetables on two dinner plates and serve.

Sweet and Sour Pork

Servings: 2 dinner entrées (four blocks each)

Block Size:

8 Protein	8 ounces pork, diced
1 Carbohydrate	2 teaspoons sugar
1 Carbohydrate	½ cup tomato puree
1 Carbohydrate	4 teaspoons cornstarch
3 Carbohydrate	1½ cups pineapple, diced
2 Carbohydrate	1 cup fruit cocktail, packed in water
8 Fat	2⅔ teaspoons olive oil

1 cup chicken stock
8 tablespoons vinegar
4 tablespoons water
2 tablespoons soy sauce
4–6 snow peas for garnish (optional)
Salt and pepper to taste

Method:
In nonstick sauté pan, cook pork in hot oil until lightly browned. While the pork is cooking, in a saucepan add chicken stock, vinegar, water, soy sauce, sugar, tomato puree, and cornstarch. (Mix cornstarch with chicken stock to dissolve cornstarch before adding to saucepan.) Simmer mixture in saucepan, stirring continuously, until it has thickened and heated through; however, do not bring mixture to a boil. Taste sauce; if it has too strong a vinegar taste, continue simmering for a few more minutes. The flavor will develop into a sweet and sour sauce as it cooks. When the desired sweet and sour sauce flavor has developed, add pork and fruit to saucepan and simmer for 10–15 minutes to allow flavors to blend and vinegar to tenderize the pork. Place an equal amount of pork and fruit on two dinner plates, garnish with snow peas, if desired, and serve.

Chicken Kabobs

Servings: 2 dinner entrées (four blocks each)

Block Size:

8 Protein	8 ounces chicken tenderloins cut into one-inch pieces (or skinless chicken breast)
2 Carbohydrate	4½ cups red bell pepper, cut in one-inch squares
2 Carbohydrate	3 cups broccoli florets
2 Carbohydrates	6 cups mushrooms, halved
2 Carbohydrate	2½ cups tomato, cubed
8 Fat	2⅔ teaspoons olive oil

2 cups chicken stock
2 tablespoons cider vinegar
⅛ teaspoon dried basil
⅛ teaspoon dried oregano
2 garlic cloves, minced
Salt and pepper to taste

Method:
Combine oil, stock, vinegar, basil, oregano, and garlic in a baking dish to create a marinade. Prepare eight skewers for kabobs. On each skewer place chicken, bell pepper, broccoli, mushrooms, and tomato, repeating the process until all ingredients have been placed on skewers. Place skewers in baking dish and baste with marinade. Tightly seal baking dish with foil. Bake in preheated oven at 350 degrees for 30 minutes. When the kabobs are ready, place four kabobs on each of the two dinner plates and serve.

Note: If you decide to grill the kabobs and are using wooden skewers, be sure to soak the sticks in water for 1 hour beforehand. Otherwise the intense heat will char them.

Chicken Marsala Forestiere

Servings: 2 dinner entrées (four blocks each)

Block Size:

8 Protein	8 ounces skinless chicken breast, diced
1 Carbohydrate	1 cup onion, sliced and halved
4 Carbohydrate	12 cups mushrooms, sliced
2 Carbohydrate	4 lemons, juice and pulp
1 Carbohydrate	4 teaspoons cornstarch
8 Fat	2⅔ teaspoons olive oil

½ cup chicken stock
2 tablespoons fresh basil, chopped
⅛ teaspoon Marsala wine
Salt and pepper to taste

Method:
In nonstick sauté pan, add oil, chicken, onion, and mushrooms. Cook until chicken and vegetables are tender, then add lemon juice and pulp, chicken stock, basil, wine, and cornstarch. (Mix cornstarch with chicken stock so that the cornstarch can dissolve before adding to pan.) Simmer ingredients in a sauté pan for 5–10 minutes, then place an equal amount of chicken and vegetables on two dinner plates and serve.

Gourmet Rock Cornish Hen à l'Orange

Servings: 2 dinner entrées (four blocks each)

Block Size:

8 Protein	1 Rock Cornish game hen, roughly 2 pounds (half of weight is in bone)
1 Carbohydrate	3 cups mushrooms, diced fine
2 Carbohydrate	2 cups onion, diced fine
2 Carbohydrate	⅔ cup mandarin orange sections
½ Carbohydrate	2 teaspoons cornstarch
1 Carbohydrate	1½ cups broccoli spears
1½ Carbohydrate	3 cups red bell pepper, diced
8 Fat	2⅔ teaspoons olive oil, divided
	4 garlic cloves, minced
	2 teaspoons parsley
	½ teaspoon paprika, divided
	½ cup chicken stock
	⅛ teaspoon white wine
	½ teaspoon orange extract
	Salt and pepper to taste

Method:
Using a large sharp knife, slice Rock Cornish hen in half along the backbone. Remove tail and skin and discard, along with gizzards. Set hen aside. In a sauté pan, add ⅔ teaspoon oil, mushrooms, garlic, parsley, and onion. Cook until mixture is translucent (about 10 minutes). (This mixture is known as a *duxell*. A duxell consists of finely cooked vegetables used to stuff another item.) When the duxell is cooked, set aside to cool. Sprinkle each Rock Cornish hen half with ¼ teaspoon paprika and rub it with remaining oil. Form two mounds of duxell in a casserole dish, place hen halves on top, and gently press them into the duxell. Tightly seal the casserole with aluminum foil and place in preheated 400-degree oven for 45 minutes. While the hen halves are cooking, combine stock, wine, orange extract, and orange sections in a small saucepan. Add cornstarch to

a little water and then stir into saucepan. Cook over medium heat until the liquid thickens to form a sauce. In another saucepan, add broccoli and bell pepper with enough water to cover. Cook until tender. Remove casserole dish from oven and drain off any juices. Using a large spatula, scoop out duxell and hen halves as one piece and place on two dinner plates. Pour orange sauce over each hen half and add an equal amount of broccoli and bell pepper to each plate. Serve immediately.

Note: This recipe takes some time to make.

Chinese Sautéed Shrimp with Tomato

Servings: 2 dinner entrées (four blocks each)

Block Size:

8 Protein	12 ounces large shrimp, cleaned, deveined, and halved (20 count)
1 Carbohydrate	2¼ cups red bell pepper, cut in quartered rings
2 Carbohydrate	2 cups snow peas, sliced in thirds
1 Carbohydrate	3 cups bean sprouts
2 Carbohydrate	2 cups scallions, chopped
2 Carbohydrate	1 cup tomato puree
8 Fat	2⅔ teaspoons olive oil

4 teaspoons ginger root, diced fine
⅛ teaspoon white wine
4 tablespoons water
2 teaspoons cider vinegar
⅛ teaspoon hot sauce
Salt and pepper to taste

Method:
In a saucepan, place bell pepper, snow peas, and sprouts in enough water to cover. Cook vegetables until they are tender. While the

vegetables are cooking, in nonstick sauté pan add oil, shrimp, and scallions. Heat shrimp and scallions until cooked, then add tomato puree, ginger root, wine, the 4 tablespoons water, vinegar, and hot sauce. Simmer for 5 minutes. On two dinner plates, arrange a bed of sprouts, snow peas, and bell peppers. Place shrimp mixture and sauce on top of vegetable mixture on both plates and serve.

Chicken Apple Pie

Servings: 2 dinner entrées (four blocks each)

Block Size:

8 Protein	8 ounces chicken tenderloins, flattened (or skinless chicken breast)
4 Carbohydrate	1⅓ cup applesauce
2 Carbohydrate	1 cup fruit cocktail, packed in water
2 Carbohydrate	6 cups mushrooms, sliced
8 Fat	2⅔ teaspoons olive oil, divided

6 tablespoons cider vinegar, divided
½ teaspoon cinnamon
⅛ teaspoon parsley
⅛ teaspoon paprika
Salt and pepper to taste

Method:
In a sauté pan, add ⅔ teaspoon oil, 4 tablespoons vinegar, and flattened chicken. Cook until chicken is browned, then add applesauce, fruit cocktail, and cinnamon to sauté pan. Simmer for 5–10 minutes to blend flavors. In a second nonstick sauté pan, add 2 teaspoons oil, 2 tablespoons vinegar, and mushrooms. Cook mushrooms until tender. On two dinner plates, place a mound of sautéed mushrooms, topped with the chicken mixture. Sprinkle with parsley and paprika and serve.

Baked Salmon

Servings: 2 dinner entrées (four blocks each)

Block Size:

8 Protein	12 ounces salmon
2 Carbohydrate	2 cups onion, sliced into rings
3 Carbohydrate	3 cups asparagus spears
1 Carbohydrate	2¼ cups red bell pepper, cut in rings
2 Carbohydrate	½ cup cooked chickpeas, chopped
8 Fat	2⅔ teaspoons olive oil

Dried dill
Garlic powder
1 cup water
Dash hot sauce (or to taste)
Dried chives
Black pepper
Celery salt

Method:
Coat bottom of a baking dish with oil, then layer the baking dish with onion rings, asparagus, bell pepper, and chickpeas. Place two fresh 6-ounce pieces of salmon on the vegetable bed in the baking dish. Sprinkle the salmon pieces lightly with dill and garlic powder, then add water and hot sauce to baking dish and seal tightly with aluminum foil. Bake in preheated oven at 350 degrees for 35 minutes. Remove baking dish from oven and drain off cooking liquid. Using a large spatula, scoop out vegetables with salmon and place on two dinner plates. Sprinkle with chives, black pepper, and celery salt, and serve.

Note: The asparagus will bleach out during cooking. If you prefer, it can be cooked separately.

Beef Roulade

Servings: 2 dinner entrées (four blocks each)

Block Size:

8 Protein	8 ounces beef eye of round, one-eighth-inch slices
1 Carbohydrate	1 cup onions, diced fine
1 Carbohydrate	½ cup carrots, diced fine
⅔ Carbohydrate	2 cups mushrooms, diced fine
1 Carbohydrate	1½ cups broccoli florets
1⅓ Carbohydrate	4 cups mushrooms, sliced
2 Carbohydrate	1 cup tomato puree
1 Carbohydrate	4 teaspoons cornstarch
8 Fat	2⅔ teaspoons olive oil
	1½ cups beef stock
	Salt and pepper to taste

Method:

Place beef slices between plastic wrap and flatten out with a mallet or heavy saucepan. In nonstick sauté pan, add oil, onions, carrots, and 2 cups diced fine mushrooms. Cook until mixture is tender. (This mixture is known as a *duxell*. A duxell consists of finely cooked vegetables used to stuff another item.) When the duxell is cooked, set aside to cool. Spoon equal amounts of the duxell mixture onto the pieces of beef and roll them up. Secure each beef roll with a wooden toothpick to form a roulade. Place rolled beef roulades, beef stock, broccoli, sliced mushrooms, tomato puree, and any leftover duxell in a medium sauté pan and cover tightly. Braise meat and vegetables in liquid for 10–15 minutes until cooked. Add a little water to the cornstarch and stir into broccoli, mushrooms, and beef stock. Heat mixture until a sauce forms, then place an equal amount of rolled beef roulades on two dinner plates, topped with vegetables and sauce.

Note: Braising is an old method of cooking that tenderizes the meat as it cooks. Usually the meat is browned in a liquid or in a covered pan on top of the stove.

Dumplings of Fish with Venetian Sauce

Servings: 2 dinner entrées (four blocks each)

Block Size:

2 Protein	4 egg whites
6 Protein	9 ounces boneless whitefish, diced
2 Carbohydrate	2½ cups tomato, diced
2 Carbohydrate	2 cups onion, diced
1 Carbohydrate	4 teaspoons cornstarch
1 Carbohydrate	1½ cups broccoli florets
2 Carbohydrate	⅔ cup applesauce

⅛ teaspoon nutmeg
1 cup water
1 cup white wine vinegar
2 tablespoons dried tarragon
⅛ teaspoon paprika
Salt and pepper to taste

Method:
A blender or food processor is needed for this recipe. Coat the bottom of a casserole dish with oil, then layer the casserole dish with the diced tomato and diced onion. Set aside for use with the fish dumplings. Place egg whites, diced raw fish, and nutmeg in a food processor. Process mixture until it forms a paste. Form fish paste into one-inch dumplings by scooping the paste into a teaspoon and placing it in a saucepan with simmering water. Hold the spoon in the simmering water for 2–3 minutes until dumpling slides off. Repeat process until all the fish paste has been used. Simmer dumpling for 4–5 minutes before removing and placing in casserole dish. In a saucepan, combine water, vinegar, and tarragon. Mix cornstarch with a little water, then add to saucepan. Simmer ingredients in saucepan for 3–5 minutes to create a Venetian sauce. Pour Venetian sauce over fish dumpling in casserole dish. Cover tightly and bake in preheated oven at 350 degrees for 15–20 minutes. While the casserole dish is in the oven, place broccoli in saucepan

with enough water to cover, and cook until tender. Remove casserole dish from oven and spoon the fish dumplings and sauce onto two dinner plates. Serve each dinner plate accompanied an equal amount of cooked broccoli and applesauce. Sprinkle with paprika and serve.

Chicken with Grapes

Servings: 2 dinner entrées (four blocks each)

Block Size:

8 Protein	8 ounces chicken tenderloins, flattened (or skinless chicken breast)
2 Carbohydrate	1½ cups red seedless grapes
2 Carbohydrate	1½ cups green seedless grapes
2 Carbohydrate	⅔ cup applesauce
1 Carbohydrate	4 teaspoons cornstarch
1 Carbohydrate	3 cups mushrooms, sliced
8 Fat	2⅔ teaspoons olive oil, divided

4 tablespoons cider vinegar, divided
2 cups plus 4 tablespoons water
2 teaspoons orange extract
⅛ teaspoon dried dill
½ teaspoon cinnamon plus ⅛ teaspoon
Dash cloves
Salt and pepper to taste

Method:
In nonstick sauté pan, add ⅔ teaspoon oil, 2 tablespoons vinegar, 2 tablespoons water, and flattened chicken. Cook until chicken is cooked. In a saucepan, place grapes, applesauce, and 2 cups water. Simmer grapes and applesauce until grapes are tender. Combine cornstarch with 2 tablespoons of water, orange extract, dill, ½ teaspoon cinnamon, and cloves to form a spicy sauce thickener. Add

spicy sauce thickener to saucepan with grapes, applesauce, and water. Cook until thickened and a grape sauce forms. Add grape sauce to chicken and simmer for 5–10 minutes to blend flavors. In another nonstick sauté pan, add 2 teaspoons oil, 2 tablespoons vinegar, ⅛ teaspoon cinnamon, and mushrooms. Cook until mushrooms are tender. On two dinner plates, place a mound of sautéed mushrooms, topped with the chicken and grape mixture.

Chicken Cacciatore

Servings: 2 dinner entrées (four blocks each)

Block Size:

8 Protein	1 pound chicken, skinless breast pieces with the bone (approximately half the weight of this chicken breast is in bone)
2 Carbohydrate	2½ cups tomato, diced
1 Carbohydrate	2¼ cups green pepper, diced
1 Carbohydrate	3 cups mushrooms, diced
1 Carbohydrate	1 cup onions, sliced
2 Carbohydrate	1 cup tomato puree
1 Carbohydrate	4 teaspoons cornstarch
8 Fat	2⅔ teaspoons olive oil
	4 garlic cloves, minced
	1 cup chicken stock
	⅛ teaspoon red wine
	1 teaspoon dried basil
	1 teaspoon dried oregano
	Salt and pepper to taste

Method:
In nonstick sauté pan, cook chicken pieces in ⅔ teaspoon oil until lightly browned. Remove chicken and place in baking dish. Using the same sauté pan, add the remaining oil, garlic, and vegetables,

except tomato puree. Cook vegetables over medium heat until tender. In saucepan, combine tomato puree, chicken stock, wine, spices, and cornstarch. (Mix cornstarch with a little water before adding to saucepan.) Cook mixture in saucepan over medium heat until a thickened sauce forms, then add vegetables to form the cacciatore sauce. Simmer sauce for 5 minutes, then place cacciatore sauce on top of chicken in baking dish. Tightly seal baking dish with aluminum foil and bake in preheated oven at 400 degrees for 20 minutes. Remove casserole dish from oven and place an equal amount of chicken on two dinner plates, topped with cacciatore sauce.

Beef à la Mode Parisienne

Servings: 2 dinner entrées (four blocks each)

Block Size:

8 Protein	8 ounces beef eye of round, one-eighth-inch slices
1 Carbohydrate	3 cups mushroom caps
2 Carbohydrate	2 cups pearl onions
2 Carbohydrate	2 cups cherry tomatoes
2 Carbohydrate	2 cups turnips, cut Parisienne style*
1 Carbohydrate	4 teaspoons cornstarch
8 Fat	2⅔ teaspoons olive oil
	2 garlic cloves, minced
	1 cup beef stock
	6 whole peppercorns
	¼ teaspoon dried oregano
	2 teaspoons fresh basil, chopped
	Salt and pepper to taste

Method:
Coat bottom of a casserole dish with oil. Place all ingredients (beef, vegetables, and spices) in medium-sized casserole dish, except basil

and cornstarch. Tightly cover casserole dish with aluminum foil and place in preheated oven at 400 degree for 20 minutes. Mix the cornstarch and basil together with a little water to form a paste. After 20 minutes, remove casserole dish from oven and stir in cornstarch-basil paste. Continue stirring meat and vegetables until they have been coated. Re-cover and cook an additional 5–10 minutes. Remove casserole dish from oven and place an equal amount of beef on two dinner plates and top with vegetables and sauce.

Note: Use a small melon ball scoop on turnips to form small balls.

Chinese Sautéed Beef and Celery

Servings: 2 dinner entrées (four blocks each)

Block Size:

8 Protein	8 ounces beef eye of round, diced fine
4 Carbohydrate	8 cups celery, willow leaf cut*
1 Carbohydrate	4 teaspoons cornstarch
1 Carbohydrate	1 kiwi fruit, sliced
2 Carbohydrate	⅔ cup mandarin orange sections
8 Fat	2⅔ teaspoons olive oil
	1 cup beef stock
	2 teaspoons red wine
	2 tablespoons low-sodium soy sauce
	2 teaspoons ginger root, diced fine

Method:

In nonstick sauté pan, add ⅔ teaspoon oil and beef. Cook beef until brown, then remove and set aside. Using the same sauté pan, add remaining oil and celery. Cook celery over medium heat until tender. While the celery is cooking, in a saucepan mix together stock, wine, soy sauce, ginger root, and cornstarch. (Mix cornstarch with cold beef stock so that the cornstarch will be dissolved before adding to saucepan.) Stir ingredients well in the saucepan, bringing to a light boil to form a sauce. Add beef and sauce to celery in sauté pan and simmer mixture for 5–10 minutes while constantly stirring beef and celery until they have been coated with sauce. Place an equal amount of beef and celery on two dinner plates, accompanied by kiwi fruit and orange sections. Serve immediately.

Note: Willow leaf cut means that the celery is cut at approximately a 45-degree angle. Also, there is no need to add any salt to this dish, because celery is naturally high in sodium.

Pizza-Topped Haddock

Servings: 2 dinner entrées (four blocks each)

Block Size:

8 Protein	12 ounces haddock
4 Carbohydrate	2 cups salsa*
4 Carbohydrate	4 cups green beans, French cut**
8 Fat	2⅔ teaspoon olive oil

Method:
Coat bottom of a baking dish with oil, then place two 6-ounce pieces of haddock in the bottom of the baking dish. Place 1 cup salsa on top of each piece of haddock. Tightly seal baking dish and bake in preheated oven at 375 degrees for 25–30 minutes. While the haddock is baking, in a saucepan add green beans and enough water to cover. Cook green beans until tender. Equally divide green beans between two dinner plates, then remove baking dish from oven. Using a large spatula, scoop out haddock and place on top of green beans on both dinner plates and serve.

Note: Salsa come with different levels of heat. Choose one that best fits your family's tastes. Someone who would like more heat than the others can add a dash of hot sauce to the portion.

**Note: If you prefer, snow peas can be substituted for the green beans.*

Salmon with Dill Sauce

Servings: 2 dinner entrées (four blocks each)

Block Size:

7 Protein	10½ ounces salmon, divided into two pieces
1 Protein and 1 Carbohydrate	½ cup plain low-fat yogurt
½ Carbohydrate	½ teaspoon sugar
½ Carbohydrate	2 teaspoons cornstarch
3 Carbohydrate	1½ cups pineapple, cubed
2 Carbohydrate	1½ cups cantaloupe, cubed
1 Carbohydrate	¾ cup maraschino cherries, halved
8 Fat	2⅔ teaspoons olive oil
	3 teaspoons dried dill weed
	2 teaspoons white wine
	Salt and pepper to taste

Method:
Coat bottom of a baking dish with oil, then place two pieces of salmon in the bottom of the baking dish. Sprinkle salmon with 1 teaspoon dill, then tightly seal baking dish and bake in preheated oven at 375 degrees for 25–30 minutes. While the salmon is baking, in a saucepan combine yogurt, sugar, 2 teaspoons dill, and wine to make the dill sauce. Add a little water to the cornstarch and then add it to dill sauce. Stirring constantly, heat sauce through but do not bring sauce to a boil. In a mixing bowl, combine pineapple, cantaloupe, and cherries to make a fruit salad. Equally divide fruit salad between two dinner plates, then remove baking dish from oven. Using a large spatula, scoop out salmon and place one piece of salmon on each dinner plate. Pour an equal amount of dill sauce over each piece of salmon and serve immediately.

Scallops Mornay

Servings: 2 dinner entrées (four blocks each)

Block Size:

6 Protein	9 ounces scallops*
2 Protein and 2 Carbohydrate	1 cup plain low-fat yogurt
3 Carbohydrate	3 cups green beans, French cut
1½ Carbohydrate	3 lemons, juice and pulp
½ Carbohydrate	½ cup onion, minced
1 Carbohydrate	4 teaspoons cornstarch
8 Fat	2⅔ teaspoons olive oil

⅛ teaspoon Worcestershire sauce
2 teaspoons dry mustard
⅛ teaspoon white wine
2 garlic cloves, minced
Paprika for garnish
Salt and pepper to taste

Method:
In nonstick sauté pan, add oil and green beans. Cook green beans until tender. While the green beans are cooking, in another nonstick sauté pan cook scallops in lemon juice with pulp, Worcestershire sauce, onion, mustard, wine, garlic, and yogurt. Cook scallops for 5–10 minutes. Depending on size of scallops, more or less cooking time may be required. Mix cornstarch with a little water and then add to scallops and simmer for 2–3 minutes until a sauce forms, stirring constantly to coat scallops. Equally divide green beans between two dinner plates. Using a serving spoon, place scallops and sauce on plates beside green beans. Serve immediately.

*Note: Small scallops are best for this dish, but if you can't find them in your supermarket or fish store, cut the larger ones into smaller pieces.

Ginger and Peach Chicken

Servings: 2 dinner entrées (four blocks each)

Block Size:

8 Protein	8 ounces chicken tenderloins, flattened (or skinless chicken breast)
4 Carbohydrate	2 cups peaches, sliced
1 Carbohydrate	½ cup water chestnuts, sliced
1 Carbohydrate	4 teaspoons cornstarch
2 Carbohydrate	2 cups snow peas
8 Fat	2⅔ teaspoons olive oil

4 tablespoons cider vinegar, divided
2 teaspoons powdered ginger*
⅛ teaspoon cinnamon, plus more
  for sprinkling
2 teaspoons orange extract
⅛ teaspoon dried dill
⅛ teaspoon cloves (scant)
1½ cups plus 4 tablespoons water

Method:
In nonstick sauté pan, add ⅔ teaspoon oil, 2 tablespoons vinegar, 2 tablespoons water, and flattened chicken. Cook until chicken is browned. In a saucepan, place peaches, ginger, and water chestnuts and 1½ cups water. Sprinkle with cinnamon. Simmer peaches until tender. Combine cornstarch with 2 tablespoons water, then add orange extract, dill weed, ⅛ teaspoon cinnamon, and cloves to form a spicy sauce thickener. Add spicy sauce thickener to saucepan with peaches and water. Cook until thickened and a peachy ginger sauce forms. Add peaches and sauce to chicken and simmer for 5–10 minutes to blend flavors and infuse chicken with ginger flavor. In another nonstick sauté pan, add 2 teaspoons oil and snow peas. Cook snow peas until tender. On two dinner plates place a mound of sautéed snow peas, topped with an equal amount of peachy ginger chicken.

Note: Adjust the amount of ginger flavor by increasing or decreasing the amount in the recipe to taste.

Antipasto Salad

Servings: 2 dinner salads (four blocks each)

Block Size:

2 Protein	2 ounces chunk light tuna*
2 Protein	2 ounces skim milk mozzarella cheese, shredded
2 Protein	3 ounces deli-style turkey, julienne
2 Protein	3 ounces deli-style ham, julienne
1 Carbohydrate	1 head iceberg lettuce, shredded
1 Carbohydrate	2 cups celery, sliced
1 Carbohydrate	½ cup carrots, sliced thin**
1 Carbohydrate	3 cups mushrooms, sliced
1 Carbohydrate	1 cup onion, in half rings
2 Carbohydrate	½ cup cooked chickpeas
1 Carbohydrate	2¼ cups red bell pepper, in half rings
8 Fat	2⅔ teaspoons extra-virgin olive oil

2 tablespoons white wine vinegar
⅛ teaspoon Worcestershire sauce
2 garlic cloves, minced
2 tablespoons water
⅛ teaspoon dried marjoram
⅛ teaspoon black pepper
⅛ teaspoon dried oregano
⅛ teaspoon dried basil

Method:

In a small mixing bowl, add oil, vinegar, Worcestershire sauce, garlic, water, and spices. Blend together with a wire whip. When finished, take two large oval plates and arrange a bed of lettuce on each plate. Place on the bed of lettuce, starting in a vertical line from the right side of the plate to the left, celery, carrots, mushrooms, onions, and chickpeas. Then place the tuna, cheese, turkey, and ham on both plates.

Divide the sections with strips of red bell pepper. Again whip herbal dressing and pour over both antipasto salads.

Note: Use water packed tuna.

**Note: Cut carrots in half and then slice thinly.*

Sautéed Beef with Mushroom Sauce

Servings: 2 dinner entrées (four blocks each)

Block Size:

8 Protein	8 ounces beef eye of round, one-eighth-inch slices
3 Carbohydrate	9 cups mushrooms, sliced
1 Carbohydrate	4 teaspoons cornstarch
3 Carbohydrate	3 cups cooked asparagus spears
1 Carbohydrate	2¼ cups red bell pepper, half rings
8 Fat	2⅔ teaspoons olive oil

1 cup beef stock
⅛ teaspoon red wine
2 garlic cloves, minced
Chopped fresh basil

Method:
In nonstick sauté pan, add ⅔ teaspoon oil and mushrooms. Cook mushrooms until tender. While the mushrooms are cooking, in another nonstick sauté pan add remaining oil and beef. Cook beef until browned, then add mushrooms, beef stock, red wine, garlic, basil, and cornstarch to sauté pan. Mix cornstarch with the beef stock before adding to the sauté pan so that the cornstarch can dissolve. Simmer, stirring frequently, until it reduces and thickens into a sauce and coats the beef. In a saucepan, add asparagus and red bell pepper with enough water to cover both vegetables. Cook until tender. On two dinner plates, equally divide the beef and vegetables. Sprinkle beef with basil and serve.

Veal Goulash

Servings: 2 dinner entrées (four blocks each)

Block Size:

8 Protein	8 ounces veal, in half-inch cubes
3 Carbohydrate	3 cups onions, diced fine
4 Carbohydrate	2 cups tomato puree
1 Carbohydrate	4 teaspoons cornstarch
8 Fat	$2\frac{2}{3}$ teaspoons olive oil

6 garlic cloves, minced
2 cups beef stock
¼ teaspoon caraway seeds
8 teaspoons paprika
4 teaspoons Worcestershire sauce
½ teaspoon celery salt
Pepper to taste
Fresh basil, roughly chopped

Method:
Coat bottom of a casserole dish with oil. Place all ingredients (veal, vegetables, and spices) in casserole dish, except basil and cornstarch. Tightly cover casserole dish with aluminum foil and place in preheated oven at 400 degrees for 20 minutes. Mix cornstarch and basil together with a little water to form a paste. Remove casserole dish from oven and stir in cornstarch-basil paste. Continue stirring meat and vegetables until they have been coated. Re-cover and cook an additional 5–10 minutes. Place an equal amount of beef pieces on two dinner plates and top with vegetables and sauce.

Mediterranean-Style Chicken

Servings: 2 dinner entrées (four blocks each)

Block Size:

8 Protein	8 ounces chicken tenderloins, flattened (or skinless chicken breast)
4 Carbohydrate	5 cups tomato, diced
4 Carbohydrate	6 cups cooked eggplant*
2 Fat	⅔ teaspoon olive oil
6 Fat	18 black olives, sliced
	8 garlic cloves, minced
	2 teaspoons dried basil
	1 teaspoon dried oregano
	4 tablespoons water
	2 tablespoons red wine

Method:

In nonstick sauté pan, add ⅔ teaspoon oil and flattened chicken. Cook chicken until lightly browned, then add diced tomato, garlic, basil, oregano, olives, water, and red wine. Simmer, covered, for 10 minutes or until almost all the liquid evaporates. While the chicken is cooking, cut eggplant in one-eighth-inch-thick slices and place in boiling salted water for 10 minutes, or until tender. On two dinner plates place a bed of cooked eggplant, then place the chicken-tomato mixture on top of the eggplant. Serve immediately.

*Note: When you are buying eggplants, look for those that are firm and have a deep purple color. The skin should have a glossy shine and be free of blemishes and discoloration.

Japanese Sweet and Sour Mandarin Shrimp

Servings: 2 dinner entrées (four blocks each)

Block Size:

8 Protein	12 ounces, cooked shrimp
1 Carbohydrate	2½ cups celery, willow leaf cut*
2 Carbohydrate	2 cups onion, rings halved
1 Carbohydrate	3 cups cucumber, peeled, halved lengthwise, and sliced
1 Carbohydrate	½ cup pineapple, diced fine
1 Carbohydrate	4 teaspoons cornstarch
2 Carbohydrate	⅔ cup mandarin orange sections**
8 Fat	2⅔ teaspoons olive oil
	8 tablespoons vinegar
	2 tablespoons soy sauce
	1 cup chicken stock
	Black pepper to taste

Method:

In nonstick sauté pan, add 2 teaspoons oil, celery, and onions. Just before the celery and onions are tender, add the cucumber. Continue cooking until all ingredients are tender. While vegetables are cooking, in small saucepan combine vinegar, soy sauce, chicken stock, shrimp, pineapple, ⅔ teaspoon oil, and cornstarch to form a sweet and sour sauce. (Mix cornstarch with a little water before adding it to saucepan, so that the cornstarch can dissolve.) Stir sweet and sour sauce until it has thickened. When the vegetables in the sauté pan are tender, add them to the sweet and sour sauce. Simmer for 2–3 minutes, then add orange sections. Divide mixture between two dinner plates and serve immediately.

*Note: Willow leaf cut means that the celery is cut at approximately a 45-degree angle. Also, there is no need to add any salt to this dish, because celery is naturally high in sodium.

**Note: Be careful not to overcook cucumber or orange sections because they will break down.

Veal Mozzarella with Italian Vegetables

Servings: 2 dinner entrées (four blocks each)

Block Size:

6 Protein	6 ounces veal scallopini
2 Protein	2 ounces skim milk mozzarella cheese, shredded
2 Carbohydrate	3 cups eggplant, half-inch cubes
2 Carbohydrate	3 cups zucchini, half-inch cubes
2 Carbohydrate	2 cups tomato, half-inch cubes
1 Carbohydrate	1 cup onions, rings halved
1 Carbohydrate	½ cup tomato puree
8 Fat	2⅔ teaspoons olive oil

2 tablespoons plus ⅛ teaspoon dried basil
⅛ teaspoon dried rosemary
½ teaspoon dried marjoram
⅛ teaspoon dried sage
⅛ teaspoon onion powder
⅛ teaspoon salt
⅛ teaspoon pepper
½ teaspoon dried oregano
4 garlic cloves, minced
½ cup plus 2 tablespoons water

Method:
In a sauté pan, add 2 teaspoons oil, spices, and vegetables, except tomato puree. Cook until tender; however, just before the vegetables are tender, add the tomato puree. While the vegetables are cooking, place veal in a second sauté pan with ⅔ teaspoon oil and 2 tablespoons water. Cook veal until browned. While the veal is cooking, sprinkle with onion powder, salt, pepper, and basil. When the veal in the sauté pan is done, divide equally between two dinner plates. Place an equal amount of vegetables on top of the veal. Lightly sprinkle both dishes with shredded mozzarella cheese and serve immediately.

Stuffed Pork Chops with Vegetable Sauce

Servings: 2 dinner entrées (four blocks each)

Block Size:

8 Protein	2 boneless pork chops (4 ounces each), trimmed
½ Carbohydrate	1½ cups mushrooms, diced fine
2 Carbohydrate	½ cup cooked chickpeas, chopped
½ Carbohydrate	½ cup onions, diced fine
1 Carbohydrate	2 cups celery, sliced
1 Carbohydrate	1½ cups broccoli, small florets or diced fine*
1 Carbohydrate	2 cups cauliflower, small florets or diced fine*
1 Carbohydrate	2¼ cups red bell pepper, medium dice
1 Carbohydrate	4 teaspoons cornstarch
8 Fat	2⅔ teaspoons olive oil
	⅛ teaspoon black pepper
	⅛ teaspoon Worcestershire sauce
	⅛ teaspoon dried marjoram
	3 cups chicken stock
	⅛ teaspoon dried basil
	⅛ teaspoon cinnamon
	⅛ teaspoon chili powder
	⅛ teaspoon nutmeg
	Salt to taste

Method:
In a sauté pan, add ⅔ teaspoon oil, mushrooms, chickpeas, black pepper, Worcestershire sauce, marjoram, and onions. Cook until mixture is translucent (about 10 minutes). (This mixture is known as a *duxell*. A duxell consists of finely cooked vegetables used to stuff another item.) When the duxell is cooked, set aside to cool. Cut a pocket in each pork chop and fill with cooled duxell. Secure pockets

with toothpicks so that the duxell will not fall out. If there is any duxell left over, then place a mound of duxell in a baking dish and place the pork chops on top of the duxell. Cover the baking dish and bake in preheated oven at 375 degrees for 20–25 minutes. While the pork chops are cooking, in saucepan combine chicken stock, celery, broccoli, cauliflower, bell pepper, basil, cinnamon, chili powder, and nutmeg. Bring to boil and cook for 10 minutes or until vegetables are tender. Mix cornstarch with a little water and add to vegetables. Reduce heat and simmer 5 minutes, until a sauce forms. Remove baking pan from oven and then carefully remove toothpicks. Place a baked pork chop on each of the two dinner plates with an equally divided amount of vegetables and sauce.

Note: Be sure that broccoli and cauliflower are in small florets or diced fine so that the vegetables will cook in the same amount of time.

Belgian Pork Chops

Servings: 2 dinner entrées (four blocks each)

Block Size:

8 Protein	8 ounces thin boneless pork chops, trimmed of fat
4 Carbohydrate	4 cups brussels sprouts*
3 Carbohydrate	3 cups onion rings, halved
1 Carbohydrate	4 teaspoons cornstarch
8 Fat	2⅔ teaspoons olive oil, divided
	2 tablespoons cider vinegar
	2 tablespoons beer
	1 cup chicken stock

Method:
In a saucepan, place brussels sprouts in enough water to cover. Cook brussels sprouts until tender. While the brussels sprouts are cooking, in a sauté pan add oil, onions, and pork chops. Cook pork chops and onions until the onions are tender and pork chops are well browned; just before the pork chops and onions are done, add 2 tablespoons cider vinegar. In another saucepan, combine beer, chicken stock, and cornstarch. (Mix cornstarch with the cold stock before adding to saucepan.) Heat beer, chicken stock, and cornstarch in saucepan until a sauce forms. When sauce has thickened, add to sauté pan with pork chops and onions, then simmer for 5–10 minutes. Place an equal amount of brussels sprouts on two dinner plates and an equal amount of pork chops and onions on each plate. Serve immediately.

*Note: Cut a cross (+) in the stem end of each brussels sprout. This helps keep them from breaking apart during the cooking process.

Broiled Lamb Chops with Basil Green Beans

Servings: 2 dinner entrées (four blocks each)

Block Size:

8 Protein	12 ounces lamb chops (approximately 4 ounces will be bone)
4 Carbohydrate	1⅓ cups unsweetened applesauce*
3 Carbohydrate	3 cups green beans
1 Carbohydrate	2¼ cups red bell pepper, quarter rings
8 Fat	2 ⅔ teaspoons olive oil

Celery salt
Onion powder
Garlic powder
Black pepper to taste
1 teaspoon fresh mint, chopped**
2 garlic cloves, minced
¼ teaspoon dried basil
2 teaspoons red bell pepper, diced fine

Method:

Sprinkle chops with celery salt, onion powder, garlic powder, and black pepper. Place them in a baking pan with a little water and broil about four inches from heat. Broil for about 5 minutes (be careful not to overcook). While the lamb chops are broiling, place the applesauce in a small saucepan, with mint and heat. In nonstick sauté pan, cook green beans and bell pepper in oil with garlic and basil. Cook until vegetables are tender. Garnish with the diced red pepper. Remove lamb chops from oven and place on two dinner plates. Place applesauce, green beans, and bell pepper beside the lamb chops and serve.

*Note: You may substitute a cored and sliced apple for the applesauce and sprinkle it with the mint.

**Note: Do not use mint extract because it overpowers the applesauce.

Braised Lamb Bretonne

Servings: 2 dinner entrées (four blocks each)

Block Size:

8 Protein	8 ounces lamb medallions, about the size of a silver dollar and one-eighth-inch thick.
4 Carbohydrate	1 cup cooked black beans
2 Carbohydrate	1 cup tomato puree
½ Carbohydrate	1 cup celery
1½ Carbohydrate	1½ cups onion, chopped fine
8 Fat	2⅔ teaspoons olive oil

2 garlic cloves, minced
⅛ teaspoon Worcestershire sauce
1 cup beef stock
⅛ teaspoon white wine
⅛ teaspoon dried basil
Salt and pepper to taste

Method:
Combine lamb and all other ingredients in a large saucepan, then cover the saucepan and simmer for 20–30 minutes. Divide between two dinner dishes and serve.

Pork Meatballs with Tomato-Tarragon Sauce

Servings: 2 dinner entrées (four blocks each)

Block Size:

8 Protein	12 ounces lean ground pork
4 Carbohydrate	1 cup cooked lentils
1 Carbohydrate	1 cup onion, diced fine
1 Carbohydrate	1½ cups steamed broccoli
2 Carbohydrate	1 cup tomato puree
8 Fat	2⅔ teaspoons olive oil

¼ teaspoon chili powder
⅛ teaspoon dried basil
⅛ teaspoon dried tarragon
⅛ teaspoon black pepper
⅛ teaspoon dried marjoram
½ cup beef stock
2 teaspoons cider vinegar

Method:
In a large mixing bowl, combine the cooked lentils, pork, diced onion, chili, basil, dash tarragon, pepper, and dash marjoram. Form mixture into 16 one-inch meatballs. Place meatballs in a baking dish brushed with oil. Bake meatballs in a preheated 375-degree oven for 15 minutes. While the meatballs are cooking, in a saucepan add broccoli and enough water to cover. Cook broccoli until tender but not overcooked. In another small saucepan, combine tomato puree, dash tarragon, dash marjoram, beef stock, and vinegar. Simmer 3–4 minutes to heat throughout. Remove meatballs from oven and gently place meatballs in sauce, gently spooning the sauce over meatballs. Place eight meatballs on each dinner plate and equally divide broccoli and serve.

Note: When a recipe calls for a dash or a pinch of an ingredient, it usually means less than ⅛ teaspoon.

Meatloaf with Italian Sauce

Servings: 2 dinner entres (four blocks each)

Block Size:

8 Protein	12 ounces ground chicken breast
1 Carbohydrate	½ cup carrots, diced fine
1 Carbohydrate	2 cups celery, diced fine
3 Carbohydrate	1½ cups tomato puree, divided
1 Carbohydrate	4 teaspoons cornstarch
8 Fat	2⅔ teaspoons olive oil

4 garlic cloves, minced
1 teaspoon dried basil, divided
1 teaspoon dried oregano, divided
Dried thyme
½ teaspoon dried marjoram
1 cup beef stock
⅛ teaspoon onion powder

Method:

In a medium bowl, mix together the chicken, carrots, celery, ½ cup tomato puree, 2 cloves garlic, ½ teaspoon basil, ½ teaspoon oregano, thyme, and marjoram. Form into two oblong meatloaves and place in baking pan. Bake in a preheated 375-degree oven for 30–35 minutes. While meatloaf is cooking, in a small saucepan combine the oil, beef stock, 1 cup puree, ½ teaspoon basil, ½ teaspoon oregano, 2 cloves garlic, onion powder, and cornstarch to make an Italian sauce. (Mix the cornstarch with the cold beef stock before adding it to the saucepan.) Lightly simmer sauce until it thickens. Remove meatloaf from oven and place on two dinner plates. The loaves are very tender. Remove from baking pan with a large spatula that will support the whole loaf. Pour Italian sauce over meatloaves and serve.

Moo Goo Gai Pan

Servings: 2 dinner entrées (four blocks each)

Block Size:

8 Protein	1 pound chicken, skinless breast pieces with the bone (approximately half the weight of this chicken breast is in bone) or 8 ounces skinless breast meat
1 Carbohydrate	3 cups mushrooms, sliced
1 Carbohydrate	1 cup scallions, sliced
1 Carbohydrate	½ cup water chestnuts, sliced
4 Carbohydrate	4 cups snow peas
1 Carbohydrate	4 teaspoons cornstarch
8 Fat	2⅔ teaspoons olive oil
	Salt
	Black pepper
	3 cups chicken stock
	2 tablespoons water
	½ teaspoon ginger root, diced fine
	2 tablespoons low-sodium soy sauce
	2 garlic cloves, minced

Method:

Sprinkle chicken with salt and pepper, then place chicken in non-stick sauté pan with 2 teaspoons oil. Cook chicken until browned and flavor has been sealed inside chicken. Place chicken in baking dish and bake in a preheated 375-degree oven for 15–20 minutes. While the chicken is cooking, in the same sauté pan used to cook the chicken, add mushrooms, scallions, and remaining oil. Cook until mushrooms and scallions are almost tender, then add chicken stock, water, water chestnuts, peapods, ginger root, soy sauce, garlic, and cornstarch. (Mix the cornstarch with a little water before adding it to the saucepan.) Heat mixture in saucepan, stirring occasionally until it is thickened. Remove chicken from oven and add chicken to mushroom-scallion sauce mixture. Coat chicken with sauce and vegetables and simmer for 3–5 minutes. Divide entrée between two dinner plates and serve.

North African Chicken Tangiers

Servings: 2 dinner entrées (four blocks each)

Block Size:

8 Protein	1 pound chicken, skinless breast pieces with the bone (approximately half the weight of chicken breast is in bone)
2 Carbohydrate	2½ cups cooked kale*
1 Carbohydrate	1½ teaspoons honey
1 Carbohydrate	4 teaspoons cornstarch
4 Carbohydrate	1⅓ cups mandarin orange sections
8 Fat	2⅔ teaspoons olive oil

Salt and pepper to taste
2 teaspoons cider vinegar
3 cups chicken stock
⅛ teaspoon red wine
¼ teaspoon ginger root, grated
½ teaspoon orange extract

Method:
Sprinkle chicken with salt and pepper, then place chicken in nonstick sauté pan with 2 teaspoons oil. Cook chicken until browned and flavor has been sealed inside chicken. Place chicken in baking dish and bake in a preheated 375-degree oven for 15–20 minutes. While the chicken is cooking in the oven, place in the nonstick sauté pan used to brown the chicken the remaining ⅔ teaspoon of oil, kale, and vinegar. Cook until kale is almost tender. In small saucepan, blend chicken stock, honey, wine, ginger root, orange extract, and cornstarch. (Mix the cornstarch with a little water before adding it to the

saucepan,) Heat mixture in saucepan, stirring occasionally until it is thickened. Remove chicken from oven and place chicken and orange sections in sauce. Do not allow orange sections to break up from overcooking. Simmer 3–5 minutes, then equally divide kale on two dinner plates and top with an equally divided amount of chicken.

Note: Kale should be just heated through, never overcooked.

Mustard Chicken

Servings: 2 dinner entrées (four blocks each)

Block Size:

6 Protein	12 ounces chicken, skinless breast pieces with the bone (approximately half the weight of chicken breast is in bone)
2 Protein and 2 Carbohydrate	1 cup plain low-fat yogurt
1 Carbohydrate	3 cups mushrooms, sliced
4 Carbohydrate	5 cups cooked kale, thickly shredded*
1 Carbohydrate	4 teaspoons cornstarch
8 Fat	2⅔ teaspoons olive oil
	Salt and pepper to taste
	1 teaspoon dry mustard
	⅛ teaspoon white wine
	½ cup chicken stock

Method:
Sprinkle chicken with salt and pepper, then place chicken in nonstick sauté pan with 2 teaspoons oil. Cook chicken until browned and flavor has been sealed inside chicken. Place chicken in baking dish and bake in a preheated 375-degree oven for 15–20 minutes. While the chicken is cooking in the oven, place in the nonstick

sauté pan used to brown the chicken the remaining ⅔ teaspoon oil, mushrooms, and kale. Cook until mushrooms and kale are almost tender. In a small saucepan, add yogurt, mustard, wine, chicken stock, and cornstarch to make a mustard sauce. (Mix the cornstarch with a little water before adding it to the saucepan.) Heat mixture in saucepan, stirring occasionally until it is thickened. Remove chicken from oven and place chicken in mustard sauce. Simmer 3–5 minutes, then equally divide mushroom-kale mixture on two dinner plates and top with an equally divided amount of chicken and mustard sauce.

Note: Kale should be just heated through, never overcooked.

Fried Deviled Chicken with Asparagus

Servings: 2 dinner entrées (four blocks each)

Block Size:

8 Protein	1 pound chicken, skinless breast pieces with the bone (approximately half the weight of chicken breast is in bone) or 8 ounces skinless breast meat
2 Carbohydrate	½ cup tomato puree
1 Carbohydrate	4 teaspoons cornstarch
2 Carbohydrate	2 cups cooked pearl onions
3 Carbohydrate	3 cups cooked asparagus
8 Fat	2⅔ teaspoons olive oil
	⅛ teaspoon paprika
	⅛ teaspoon dried basil
	⅛ teaspoon onion powder
	⅛ teaspoon garlic powder
	⅛ teaspoon dried oregano
	Salt and pepper to taste
	2 garlic cloves, minced
	1 cup chicken stock

½ teaspoon hot curry powder
¼ teaspoon white pepper
Water

Method:
Sprinkle chicken with paprika, basil, onion powder, garlic powder, oregano, salt, and pepper, then place chicken in nonstick sauté pan with 2 teaspoons oil. Cook chicken until browned and flavor has been sealed inside chicken. Place chicken in baking dish and bake in a preheated 375-degree oven for 15–20 minutes. While the chicken is cooking in the oven, place in the nonstick sauté pan used to brown the chicken the remaining ⅔ teaspoon oil, tomato puree, minced garlic, chicken stock, curry powder, pepper, and cornstarch. Blend cornstarch with a little water before adding to sauté pan. Simmer for 5–10 minutes to blend flavors and allow mixture to thicken into a sauce, then add pearl onions. In a saucepan, add asparagus and enough water to cover. Cook asparagus until tender but not overcooked. Remove chicken from oven and place chicken in sauté pan. Coat chicken with sauce while simmering for an additional 5 minutes. Equally divide asparagus on two dinner plates and place equally divided amount of chicken and devil sauce on plate.

Braised Pork and Cabbage

Servings: 2 dinner entrées (four blocks each)

Block Size:

8 Protein	12 ounces ground pork
3 Carbohydrate	9 cups cabbage, shredded
2 Carbohydrate	½ cup chickpeas, chopped
1 Carbohydrate	3 cups mushrooms, sliced
2 Carbohydrate	4 teaspoons granulated sugar
8 Fat	2⅔ teaspoons olive oil
	¼ teaspoon black pepper
	⅛ teaspoon celery salt

8 tablespoons cider vinegar
1 cup chicken stock
¼ teaspoon marjoram
⅛ teaspoon caraway seed
Paprika

Method:

In a small mixing bowl, sprinkle pork with pepper and celery salt and mix throughout. In a medium-sized nonstick sauté pan, cook pork in ⅔ teaspoon oil over medium-high heat until browned. While the pork is cooking, in another nonstick sauté pan add remaining oil, cabbage, chickpeas, mushrooms, vinegar, sugar, and other spices. Cook vegetable mixture for about 10–15 minutes, until vegetables are almost tender, then add stock and cooked pork to the sauté pan. Braise mixture for 5–10 minutes, until heated through. Divide between two dinner dishes and serve with paprika sprinkled on top.

Chicken Gumbo Creole

Servings: 2 dinner entrées (four blocks each)

Block Size:

8 Protein	8 ounces chicken tenderloins, diced (or skinless chicken breast)
1 Carbohydrate	2 cups celery, diced fine
2 Carbohydrate	2 cups onion, diced fine
1 Carbohydrate	1¼ cups tomato, diced fine
1 Carbohydrate	2¼ cups green peppers, diced fine
1 Carbohydrate	1 cup okra, cut in half-inch slices
2 Carbohydrate	⅔ cup cooked long-grain rice*
8 Fat	2⅔ teaspoons olive oil
	¼ teaspoon tabasco sauce or to taste
	2 garlic cloves, minced
	3 cups chicken stock**

Method:
Combine diced chicken and all ingredients together in a mixing bowl. Mix gently, then place the mixture in a large saucepan. Cover the saucepan and simmer on medium-high heat for 25–30 minutes. Divide into two soup bowls and serve.

*Note: ⅖ cup is approximately halfway between ⅓ and ½ cup.

**Note: If a thinner soup is desired, add 2 more cups stock.

Beefy-Vegetable Stir-Fry

Servings: 2 dinner entrées (four blocks each)

Block Size:

8 Protein	12 ounces lean ground beef
2 Carbohydrate	2 cups onion, sliced and halved
3 Carbohydrate	¾ cup chickpeas, rinsed and chopped
1 Carbohydrate	1½ cups red bell pepper, sliced and quartered
1 Carbohydrate	3 cups cabbage, shredded
1 Carbohydrate	3 cups mushrooms, sliced
8 Fat	2⅔ teaspoon olive oil, divided
	2 tablespoons apple cider vinegar
	¼ teaspoon Worcestershire sauce
	Salt and pepper to taste
	1 tablespoon low-sodium soy sauce

Method:
In nonstick sauté pan, add ground beef, onion, and ⅔ teaspoon oil. Cook ground beef and onion until browned. In another nonstick sauté pan, add 2 teaspoons oil and remaining ingredients, and cook until cabbage is tender. When the cabbage is tender, add cooked beef and onions to the cabbage. Simmer entire mixture for 10–15 minutes. Divide mixture between two dinner plates and serve.

Tangy Chicken and Bean Salad

Servings: 2 dinner entrées (four blocks each)

Block Size:

8 Protein	8 ounces chicken tenderloins, diced (or skinless chicken breast)
1 Carbohydrate	1 cup fresh green beans, half-inch pieces
1 Carbohydrate	¼ cup cooked red kidney beans, rinsed
1 Carbohydrate	1 cup onion, diced fine
1 Carbohydrate	¼ cup chickpeas, rinsed
½ Carbohydrate	½ head lettuce, shredded
1 Carbohydrate	1¼ cups tomato, diced
½ Carbohydrate	1½ cups raw mushrooms, sliced
1 Carbohydrate	1 cucumber, peeled, seeded, diced
1 Carbohydrate	6 cups spinach
8 Fat	2⅔ teaspoons olive oil

¼ cup water
¼ cup apple cider vinegar
⅛ teaspoon dry mustard
⅛ teaspoon cayenne pepper
⅛ teaspoon chili powder
⅛ teaspoon curry powder (Madras hot)
¼ teaspoon celery salt

Method:

In medium-sized sauté pan, add 2 teaspoons oil, chicken, green beans, kidney beans, onion, and chickpeas. Cook on medium-high heat for 10–15 minutes until the chicken is done and vegetables are crispy-tender. While the chicken and vegetables are cooking, in a saucepan add ⅔ teaspoon oil, water, vinegar, and spices, and heat.

When the mixture in the saucepan has come to a boil, add liquid to the chicken and vegetables and stir to coat the chicken and vegetables. On two large dinner plates, arrange a bed of lettuce, tomato, mushrooms, cucumber, and spinach to form a salad. Top the salad with the chicken mixture and serve.

SNACKS AND DESSERTS

Jellied Fruit Salad with Walnuts

Servings: 4 serving dishes (one block each)

Block Size:

4 Protein	4 envelopes Knox Unflavored Gelatin
1 Carbohydrate	1 kiwi fruit, peeled and diced
1 Carbohydrate	1 cup raspberries
1 Carbohydrate	1 cup strawberries, diced
1 Carbohydrate	½ cup seedless red grapes, halved
4 Fat	4 teaspoons walnuts, chopped
	2 cups water
	1 tablespoon banana extract
	1 tablespoon orange extract
	½ teaspoon strawberry extract
	Mint leaves

Method:

In saucepan, place gelatin and water, stir until dissolved, then add fruit and extracts. Heat to a simmer, stirring gently for 10 minutes until the raspberries dissolve. Pour liquid into eight-inch by eight-inch by two-inch pan and let cool. When Jellied Fruit Salad has set, place in four serving dishes and garnish with mint leaves.

Note: When choosing berries, look for those that are medium-sized and uniform in color. They should also feel solid to the touch and not be leaking juice.

Orange-Yogurt Dessert

Servings: 4 serving dishes (one block each)

Block Size:

1 Protein	1 envelope Knox Unflavored Gelatin
1 Protein	3 ounces extra-firm tofu, mashed
2 Protein and 2 Carbohydrate	1 cup plain low-fat yogurt
2 Carbohydrate	⅔ cup mandarin orange sections
4 Fat	1⅓ teaspoons olive oil
	1 teaspoon orange extract
	¼ teaspoon cinnamon
	Mint leaves

Method:

In saucepan, place gelatin, yogurt, tofu, and oil, stir until gelatin is dissolved, then add fruit, orange extract, and mint leaves. Heat to a simmer, stirring gently, for 10 minutes until orange sections start to break down. Pour into eight-inch by eight-inch by two-inch pan and let cool. When orange-yogurt has set, cut into cubes and place in four serving dishes. Sprinkle orange-yogurt cubes with cinnamon before serving.

Note: When using yogurt in a recipe, be sure not to bring it to a boil. This will cause the yogurt to break down. This can also happen if it is stirred too much.

Apple-Cinnamon Squares

Servings: 4 serving dishes (one block each)

Block Size:

4 Protein	4 envelopes Knox Unflavored Gelatin
4 Carbohydrate	1⅓ cups applesauce
4 Fat	1⅓ teaspoons olive oil
	2 cups water
	⅛ teaspoon nutmeg
	1 teaspoon cinnamon

Method:
In saucepan, place 2 cups water, gelatin, and oil, stir until gelatin is dissolved, then add applesauce, nutmeg, and cinnamon. Heat to a simmer, stirring gently for 10 minutes. Pour into eight-inch by eight-inch by two-inch pan and let cool. When Apple-Cinnamon Squares have set, cut into cubes and place on four serving dishes.

Melon Wrapped in Ham

Servings: 4 serving dishes (one block each)

Block Size:

4 Protein	6 ounces deli-style ham, cut in strips
4 Carbohydrate	1 cantaloupe, quartered and cubed*
4 Fat	12 black olives

Method:
Wrap ham around melon cubes and secure with a toothpick. Arrange on serving dish and garnish with olives.

*Note: For a more elegant presentation, use a large melon ball scoop instead of cubing the melon.

Dessert Omelette

Servings: 8 serving dishes (one block each)

Block Size:

8 Protein	14 egg whites plus 2 egg yolks (separate egg whites from yolks)
2 Carbohydrate	4 teaspoons granulated sugar
3 Carbohydrate	3 cups strawberries, sliced
3 Carbohydrate	1 cup mandarin orange sections
8 Fat	2⅔ teaspoons olive oil
	Pinch salt

Method:
In a medium-sized mixing bowl, whip egg whites to form a meringue (marshmallowlike consistency). In another bowl, beat egg yolks, sugar, and pinch of salt. Gently pour egg yolks into meringue and fold in with a spatula until it becomes marbleized. Heat oil in a medium sauté pan, then pour the egg mixture into the sauté pan and smooth it out into an even layer. On medium-high heat, cook until the edges of the egg mixture are dry and the center is somewhat creamy. Lift the edge of the omelette in the pan to check the color; it should be a light golden brown color. Remove from heat and place under a broiler until center is set. As soon as the omelette has set, remove from broiler and spoon some of the strawberries in a line along the center. Add the rest of the strawberries and the mandarin oranges to the omelette and fold over the other half. Remove the omelette from the pan and transfer to a plate. Cut the omelette into eight portions and place on serving dishes.

Frozen Peach Yogurt

Servings: 8 serving dishes (one block each)

Block Size:

3 Protein	3 envelopes Knox Unflavored Gelatin
1 Protein	2 egg whites
4 Protein and 4 Carbohydrate	2 cups plain low-fat yogurt
3 Carbohydrate	3 peaches, halved, pitted, and chopped
1 Carbohydrate	2 teaspoons sugar
8 Fat	8 teaspoons slivered almonds
	2 teaspoons vanilla extract
	⅛ teaspoon ginger
	Dash allspice

Method:

In saucepan, place yogurt, gelatin, fruit, spices, and extract. Heat until mixture becomes thoroughly warm, no more than 180 degrees. Cool and set aside. In a mixing bowl, whip egg whites until firm. When the mixture in the saucepan has cooled, combine it with the whipped egg whites and chopped almonds. Place mixture in a pan and place in freezer or add mixture to an ice cream maker and blend. When mixture is frozen, scoop into eight small serving dishes.

Frozen Strawberry Yogurt

Servings: 8 serving dishes (one block each)

Block Size:

3 Protein	3 envelopes Knox Unflavored Gelatin
1 Protein	2 egg whites
4 Protein and 4 Carbohydrate	2 cups plain low-fat yogurt
3 Carbohydrate	3 cups strawberries, diced fine
1 Carbohydrate	2 teaspoons sugar
8 Fat	8 teaspoons almonds, chopped fine
	2 teaspoons imitation strawberry extract

Method:

In saucepan, place yogurt, gelatin, fruit, and extract. Heat until mixture becomes thoroughly warm, no more than 180 degrees. Cool and set aside. In a mixing bowl, whip egg whites and sugar until firm. When the mixture in the saucepan has cooled, combine it with the whipped egg whites and chopped almonds. Place mixture in pan and place in freezer or add mixture to an ice cream maker and blend. When mixture is frozen, scoop into eight small serving dishes.

Frozen Orange Cream

Servings: 8 serving dishes (one block each)

Block Size:

3 Protein	3 envelopes Knox Unflavored Gelatin
1 Protein	2 egg whites
4 Protein and 4 Carbohydrate	2 cups plain low-fat yogurt
3 Carbohydrate	1 cup mandarin orange sections
1 Carbohydrate	2 teaspoons sugar
8 Fat	8 teaspoon almonds, chopped fine
	⅛ teaspoon cinnamon
	2 teaspoons orange extract

Method:

In saucepan, place yogurt, gelatin, fruit, cinnamon, and extract. Heat until mixture becomes thoroughly warm, no more than 180 degrees. Cool and set aside. In a mixing bowl, whip egg whites until firm. When the mixture in the saucepan has cooled, combine it with the whipped egg whites and chopped almonds. Place mixture in a pan and place in freezer or add mixture to an ice cream maker and blend. When mixture is frozen, scoop into eight small serving dishes.

Cottage Cheese Pudding

Servings: 8 serving dishes (one block each)

Block Size:

1 Protein	1 envelope Knox Unflavored Gelatin
1½ Protein	1 egg plus 1 egg white
4 Protein	1 cup low-fat cottage cheese
½ Protein and	
½ Carbohydrate	¼ cup plain low-fat yogurt
1 Protein and	
1 Carbohydrate	1 cup 1 percent milk
1 Carbohydrate	2 teaspoons sugar
1 Carbohydrate	¾ cup maraschino cherries
4½ Carbohydrate	2¼ cups fruit cocktail
8 Fat	8 teaspoons slivered almonds

Method:

In saucepan, combine gelatin, yogurt, milk, egg, and egg white. Heat mixture in saucepan while constantly stirring, until heated to just below boiling. Remove from heat and cool for 5 minutes before stirring in the remaining ingredients. Pour into eight dessert dishes and let set.

Strawberry Soufflé

Servings: 4 serving dishes

Block Size:

1 Protein	1 envelope Knox Unflavored Gelatin
3 Protein	6 egg whites
2 Carbohydrate	2 cups strawberries, pureed* (makes 1 cup)
1 Carbohydrate	1 lemon, pulp and juice
1 Carbohydrate	2 teaspoons sugar
4 Fat	1⅓ teaspoons olive oil
	Cream of tartar

Method:
In a medium-sized mixing bowl, whip egg whites and cream of tartar to form a meringue (marshmallowlike consistency). Place bowl to one side while preparing puree filling. Place strawberries, gelatin, lemon, and sugar in saucepan and heat until hot. Cool strawberry mixture for about 5 minutes, then pour the puree into the whipped egg whites. Gently fold strawberry puree into whipped egg whites until mixture is uniform in color. Spoon the batter into four soufflé dishes that have been brushed with the 1⅓ teaspoons oil. (If you prefer, you can add mixture to a two-quart soufflé dish, and then divide into four serving dishes after it is removed from the oven. However, individual soufflé dishes make a nice presentation.) Level off the top of the batter in the soufflé dishes. When filling the soufflé dishes, fill to only about a quarter inch from rim of dish. This will ensure that the soufflé will form properly. Bake the soufflé dishes in a preheated 375-degree oven for 20 minutes, or until the soufflé is puffed and lightly browned. Serve at once.

*Note: Any berry in season may be substituted.

Fruit Salad

Servings: 4 serving dishes (one block each)

Block Size:

4 Protein	1 cup low-fat cottage cheese
1 Carbohydrate	⅓ cup mandarin orange sections*
1 Carbohydrate	½ apple, peeled, cored, and chopped
1 Carbohydrate	1 kiwi fruit, peeled and chopped*
1 Carbohydrate	1 cup raspberries*
4 Fat	4 crushed macadamia nuts
	Fresh ground black pepper to taste Cinnamon

Method:
In a mixing bowl, combine pepper and cottage cheese, blend thoroughly, then place a small mound of peppered cottage cheese on four serving plates. In another mixing bowl, mix all fruits together to form a fruit salad. Place fruit salad around cottage cheese on four serving plates. Sprinkle with crushed macadamia nuts and cinnamon and serve.

Note: Any other fruits in season can be substituted, as long as the blocks remain the same.

Fruit Curry

Servings: 4 serving dishes (one block each)

Block Size:

4 Protein	1 cup low-fat cottage cheese
¼ Carbohydrate	½ teaspoon granulated sugar
¼ Carbohydrate	¼ teaspoon brown sugar
¼ Carbohydrate	½ lemon, pulp and juice*
½ Carbohydrate	2 teaspoons cornstarch
½ Carbohydrate	¼ cup pineapple, cubed
1 Carbohydrate	¾ cup peaches, chopped
¾ Carbohydrate	¾ kiwi fruit, peeled and chopped
½ Carbohydrate	½ cup strawberries, quartered
3 Fat	1 teaspoon olive oil
1 Fat	1 teaspoon slivered almonds, toasted

2 tablespoons water
Dash rum
¼ teaspoon cinnamon
¼ teaspoon ginger
Dash curry
Dash nutmeg
Cocoa powder
Fresh mint leaves, chopped

Method:

In a sauté pan, place 2 tablespoons water, oil, sugars, lemon pulp and juice, rum, cinnamon, ginger, curry, nutmeg, and cornstarch. (Mix cornstarch with a little water and then add to sauté pan.) Cook mixture on medium-high heat, stirring constantly until a saucelike consistency forms. Add fruit and continue cooking for 3–4 minutes. Mound cottage cheese in the center of four serving plates. When the fruit is heated through, spoon fruit around cheese on serving plates. Sprinkle with almonds, cocoa powder, and mint.

*Note: Choose lemons that are a solid yellow color. The skins should be thin and smooth. It is best to store lemons at room temperature.

Yogurt-Sauced Peaches

Servings: 4 serving dishes (one block each)

Block Size:

2 Protein	½ cup cottage cheese
2 Protein and 2 Carbohydrate	1 cup plain low-fat yogurt
2 Carbohydrate	1½ cups peaches, chunks
4 Fat	4 teaspoons almonds, chopped
	⅛ teaspoon cardamom

Method:
Using a blender, combine cottage cheese and cardamom. Blend until mixture is smooth. Fold yogurt into blended cottage cheese to make a spiced yogurt sauce. Divide peaches into four serving dishes. Spoon sauce over peaches and sprinkle with almonds. Chill and serve.

Stuffed Tomato Snacks

Servings: 4 serving dishes (one block each)

Block Size:

4 Protein	1 cup low-fat cottage cheese
3 Carbohydrate	4 tomatoes, halved and pulp removed
1 Carbohydrate	1 cucumber, peeled, seeded, and shredded
4 Fat	4 teaspoons almonds, chopped
	Salt and pepper to taste
	⅛ teaspoon dried dill
	⅛ teaspoon paprika

Method:

Using a knife, cut tomatoes in half, then carefully cut out the insides of the tomatoes to create tomato shells. Sprinkle insides of tomatoes with salt and pepper. Dice tomato pulp into small chunks. In a mixing bowl, combine cottage cheese, diced tomato chunks, chopped almonds, dill, salt, pepper, and shredded cucumber. Place two tomato shells on each of the four serving plates, then stuff tomatoes with cheese mixture and let any excess cheese mixture overflow tomato shell onto each plate. Sprinkle with paprika and cover dishes with plastic wrap. Chill before serving.

Vegetables with Garden Dip

Servings: 4 serving dishes (one block each)

Block Size:

3 Protein	¾ cup low-fat cottage cheese
1 Protein and 1 Carbohydrate	½ cup plain low-fat yogurt
1 Carbohydrate	1½ cups broccoli florets
1 Carbohydrate	2 cups cauliflower florets
1 Carbohydrate	2 cups celery sticks
4 Fat	4 teaspoons almonds, chopped
	⅛ teaspoon garlic powder
	1 tablespoon parsley
	1 teaspoon chives
	1 teaspoon chili powder
	1 teaspoon basil
	Hot sauce to taste

Method:

In medium bowl, gently combine cottage cheese, yogurt, almonds, and seasonings. Pour blended mixture into four serving bowls on a lunch plate. Place washed raw vegetables on lunch plate around serving bowls and serve.

Sweetened Peaches

Servings: 4 serving dishes (one block each)

Block Size:

4 Protein   1 cup low-fat cottage cheese

1 Carbohydrate   2 teaspoons sugar
3 Carbohydrate   2¼ cups canned peaches, sliced

4 Fat   1⅓ teaspoons olive oil

                             5 tablespoons water

Method:
In nonstick sauté pan, heat oil and sugar, continuously stirring until sugar melts. When sugar has melted, add peaches and stir to coat peaches with sugar. Add 3 tablespoons water and stir occasionally to loosen peaches. Cook peaches until they are lightly browned on all sides. While peaches are cooking, place cottage cheese in four serving dishes. Remove peaches from pan and add on top of cottage cheese. Add 2 more tablespoons water to the sauté pan and heat water until it deglazes the pan and forms a thin sauce. Pour over peaches.

Spiced Caramelized Apples

Servings: 4 serving dishes (one block each)

Block Size:

4 Protein	1 cup low-fat cottage cheese
1 Carbohydrate	2 teaspoons sugar
3 Carbohydrate	1½ apples, peeled, cored, and chopped*
4 Fat	1⅓ teaspoons olive oil
	⅛ teaspoon allspice
	¼ teaspoon cinnamon
	Dash nutmeg
	5 tablespoons water

Method:

In a sauté pan, heat oil and sugar, stirring continuously until sugar melts. When sugar has melted, add apples and spices, stir to coat apples. Add 3 tablespoons water and stir occasionally to loosen apples. Cook apples until they are lightly browned on all sides. While apples are cooking, place cottage cheese in four serving dishes. Remove apples from pan and add on top of cottage cheese. Add 2 tablespoons water to the sauté pan. Cook liquid until it forms a thin sauce. Pour over apples.

*Note: To stop apples from turning brown, dip cut apples in a little lemon juice and water mixture.

Strawberry-Yogurt Jelly

Servings: 4 serving dishes (one block each)

Block Size:

2 Protein	2 envelopes Knox Unflavored Gelatin
2 Protein and 2 Carbohydrate	1 cup plain low-fat yogurt
1 Carbohydrate	2 teaspoons granulated sugar
1 Carbohydrate	1 cup strawberries, hulled and pureed
4 Fat	4 macadamia nuts, crushed
	½ cup water

Method:
In saucepan, place gelatin and water, stirring until dissolved. Heat gelatin and water over low heat, bringing mixture to a simmer, then remove from heat and cool to room temperature. In a mixing bowl, combine yogurt, sugar, and strawberries. When the gelatin has cooled to room temperature, add yogurt mixture and stir until uniform. Pour into four serving glasses and refrigerate until set (about two hours). Sprinkle macadamia nuts evenly over the four glasses before serving.

Stuffed Melon

Servings: 4 serving dishes (one block each)

Block Size:

4 Protein	1 cup low-fat cottage cheese
1 Carbohydrate	½ cup melon balls, from two fresh melons*
1 Carbohydrate	¾ cup peach chunks
1 Carbohydrate	¾ cup maraschino cherries
1 Carbohydrate	⅓ cup mandarin orange sections
4 Fat	4 teaspoons slivered almonds

Method:
Cut 2 small melons in half to form four melon bowls. If necessary, cut the ends of the melons so that the melon bowls will sit on a plate without moving. Using a melon baller, remove the flesh by scooping out the melon. Leave a thin border wall inside the melon bowls. Mound cottage cheese in the center of each melon shell. In a mixing bowl combine fruits, then equally divide fruit and spoon on top of cottage cheese in melon bowls. Garnish with almonds and serve.

*Note: Depending on the size of the melon, you may not need all the flesh from two melons, so store the excess or use in another recipe.

Zucchini Dip

Servings: 4 serving dishes (one block each)

Block Size:

4 Protein	1 cup low-fat cottage cheese
2 Carbohydrate	2½ cups steamed zucchini, chopped
1 Carbohydrate	1½ cups broccoli florets
1 Carbohydrate	2 cups cauliflower florets
1 Fat	2 teaspoons imitation bacon bits
3 Fat	3 teaspoons slivered almonds

⅛ teaspoon dried basil
Salt and pepper to taste
Dash garlic powder
⅛ teaspoon nutmeg
⅛ teaspoon chives

Method:
In saucepan, place zucchini and enough water to cover. Cook until tender. Remove from stove and cool. Using a blender, combine cooked zucchini, cottage cheese, and spices. Blend until mixture is smooth, fold in bacon bits and slivered almonds, and scoop into four serving bowls. Arrange an equal amount of washed fresh broccoli and cauliflower florets around dip. Chill and serve.

Tomato-Zucchini Nibbles

Servings: 4 serving dishes (one block each)

Block Size:

4 Protein	1 cup cottage cheese
1 Carbohydrate	1¼ cups zucchini, chopped fine
3 Carbohydrate	3 cups cherry tomatoes
4 Fat	4 teaspoons slivered almonds, chopped
	¼ teaspoon garlic salt
	1 teaspoon snipped chives

Method:

In saucepan, place zucchini and enough water to cover. Cook until tender. Remove from stove and cool. Using a knife, cut the tomatoes in half, then carefully cut out the inside of the tomato or use a small melon baller to scoop out the inside of the tomato to create a tomato shell. If necessary, cut a little off the bottom of the tomatoes so that the tomatoes will sit on a plate without moving. Using a blender, combine cooked zucchini, tomato pulp, cottage cheese, almonds, garlic salt, and chives. Blend until mixture is smooth. Fill tomatoes with cheese mixture by piping it out with a pastry bag. Arrange on serving plates and chill.

Yogurt-Berry Bowl

Servings: 4 serving dishes (one block each)

Block Size:

4 Protein	2 cups plain low-fat yogurt
2 Carbohydrate	1 cup blueberries
1 Carbohydrate	1 cup raspberries
1 Carbohydrate	1 cup strawberries, sliced
4 Fat	4 teaspoons slivered almonds

Method:
In a mixing bowl, combine all ingredients except almonds and gently blend. Equally divide into four portions, sprinkle with almonds, and chill before serving.

Afternoon Fruity–Cottage Cheese Snack

Servings: 4 serving dishes (one block each)

Block Size:

4 Protein	1 cup low-fat cottage cheese
1 Carbohydrate	¾ cup cantaloupe, cubed
1 Carbohydrate	½ cup honeydew melon, cubed
1 Carbohydrate	¾ cup canned peaches, cubed
1 Carbohydrate	½ cup pineapple, cubed
4 Fat	4 teaspoons slivered almonds

Method:
Place ¼ cup cottage cheese in a mound in the center of four serving dishes. Surround the cottage cheese with fruit cubes and sprinkle with almonds.

10

SHOPPING IN THE WAR ZONE

It's a war out there. In fact, every time you enter the supermarket, consider it a war zone. It's you versus the food industry. And it's not fair. The food manufacturers have the high-tech weapons (e.g., marketing and packaging). You don't. They have the resources (e.g., advertising). You don't. The only thing you have in your favor is knowledge. Put that knowledge to work, and you can win the battle and the war.

First things first. Before you go off to battle, make sure that you're prepared. Eat a Zone snack before you shop. When you get to the store, follow this ideal battle plan: Try to stay on the periphery of the supermarket and never go down the aisles. Once you venture within, it's like a scene from *Moby Dick* in which Ahab is beckoning you to go after all of those neatly packaged carbohydrates and take them home to eat. Although Ahab's crew was powerless to prevent their doom, you don't have to be.

For once, the government is finally on your side in this battle of wits. Those nutritional labels that once seemed so meaningless give you the information you need to make intelligent choices in the trenches. Let's take a close look at what is commonly seen as another government make-work intervention in your life: the nutrition panel label. When people look at a nutrition panel label (see Figure 10-1), most see only one thing: the dreaded grams of FAT.

If you've read this far, you know that fat is not your enemy (and in fact it may be your greatest ally in getting into the Zone). In fact,

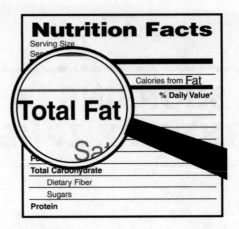

Figure 10-1. Nutritional Panel

within the borders of the nutritional label lies the real information that's going to allow you to win this war. And what is that information? The ratio of protein to carbohydrate in that food product.

That's right, every packaged food in America contains the real information you need to win the Zone war. For every 3 grams of protein, you want about 4 grams of carbohydrate. Let's be frank. It is highly unlikely that you will ever find a single food product in those aisles that has the right protein-to-carbohydrate ratio. The secret is to mix and match foods until you get the right combination. If you are going to do this mixing and matching within the confines of the supermarket, you have to go back to the blocks. Simply convert every label into blocks (divide the number of protein grams per serving by 7 grams and the number of carbohydrate grams per serving by 9 grams) and you can quickly tell what other kinds of food you need to buy to keep a precise balance in your hormonal carburetor.

For example, let's read the label on one of the first convenience foods introduced into America—Grape-Nuts. What seems more all-American than Grape-Nuts? I know this all too well. As a young high school athlete, I lived on Grape-Nuts. Grape-Nuts for breakfast, Grape-Nuts for after-school snacks, Grape-Nuts for dinner (I didn't particularly like vegetables or low-fat protein), Grape-Nuts for a late-night snack. But what was I really eating? Sugar, and lots of it. Let's look at the label. Figure 10-2 shows a Grape-Nuts nutritional label.

Nutrition Facts

Serving Size 1/2 cup
Servings 8

Amount Per Serving

Calories 200	Calories from Fat 10

% Daily Value*

Total Fat 1g

Saturated Fat 0g

Cholesterol 0mg

Sodium 350mg

Potassium   mg

Total Carbohydrate 47g

Dietary Fiber 5g

Sugars 7g

Protein 6g

Figure 10-2. Grape-Nuts Label

A ½-cup serving (2 ounces) has 6 grams of protein and 47 grams of carbohydrate. But since it also has 5 grams of fiber, the total content of insulin-promoting carbohydrate is only 42 grams. Of course, no one ever eats only 1 ounce of Grape-Nuts (more likely about 4 ounces, since that is what it takes to fill a typical bowl). Nonetheless, whether I ate 1 ounce or 4 ounces, the protein-to-carbohydrate ratio, and hence the effect on my hormonal carburetor, would be the same.

Let's assume that I ate my typical 4-ounce serving. In that serving I should be getting 12 grams of protein, but because of the fiber content, I will actually absorb less than that listed amount of protein. Let's assume that only 75 percent is absorbed (which is typical of most nonanimal sources of protein), which means that in a 4-ounce serving, I would actually be getting 9 grams of protein. Take that 9 grams of protein and divide it by 84 grams of carbohydrate, which gives a protein-to-carbohydrate ratio of 0.11. Since you are trying to get 3 grams of protein for every 4 grams of carbohydrate (a protein-to-carbohydrate ratio of 0.75), a bowl of Grape-Nuts is definitely not going to put you in the Zone.

In fact, the protein-to-carbohydrate ratio of Grape-Nuts is actually very similar to a typical candy bar. Even adding a little milk to it would not greatly change the ratio. No wonder I never made it to the NBA.

But a far better way to calculate is to break the Grape-Nuts into blocks. So let's look at the typical 4-ounce bowl of Grape-Nuts in blocks. Nine grams of protein is a little more than one protein block (9 grams of absorbed protein divided by 7 grams of protein per block). Eighty-four grams of total carbohydrate is approximately nine blocks of carbohydrates (84 grams of total carbohydrate divided by 9 grams of carbohydrate per block). What's wrong with this picture? First, the ratio of protein-to-carbohydrate blocks is nowhere near the 1:1 ratio needed for your hormonal carburetor. Second, you are consuming far more carbohydrate blocks than even the largest person would ever want in a meal. Third, there are no fat blocks. Summation, a hormonal disaster, but a correctable hormonal disaster. Simply eat less Grape-Nuts (like 1 ounce, which would give you three carbohydrate blocks) with a little low-fat milk, add another three blocks of low-fat protein (like ¾ cup of nonfat cottage cheese) and three blocks of fat using three macadamia nuts. Now you have the makings of a hormonal winner. Of course, an even better choice would have been to replace the Grape-Nuts completely with one cup of strawberries and an orange. But we're winning the battle.

Let's try looking at a typical 6-ounce can of tuna fish.

Each serving contains 12 grams of protein, 5 grams of fat, and zero grams of carbohydrate. So we have two blocks of protein per serving (12 grams divided by 7 grams equals approximately two blocks), two blocks of internal fat (5 grams divided by the 1.5 grams in one fat block equals approximately three blocks), and zero carbohydrate.

Nutrition Facts

Serving Size 2oz.
Servings 2.5

Amount Per Serving

Calories 95   Calories from Fat 45

% **Daily Value***

Total Fat 5g

Saturated Fat 2g

Cholesterol 35mg

Sodium 250mg

Potassium   mg

Total Carbohydrate 0g

Dietary Fiber 0g

Sugars 0g

Protein 12g

Figure 10-3. Label of Canned Tuna Fish

Here's an example of hidden fat found in all low-fat protein sources. Every block of low-fat protein will contain about one block of fat. That internal fat is not quite enough to optimize your hormonal carburetor. To do so, you should add one additional external block of fat for every block of low-fat protein. Now if you add up the internal fat in the low-fat protein and the external fat you plan to add, you will get the appropriate balance of protein, carbohydrate, and fat.

However, nobody eats half a can of tuna, so let's try and decipher the label of a whole can to see that each can contains about three servings. So a whole can of tuna fish would contain six protein blocks, and no carbohydrate. Obviously, if you are going to have a can of tuna for a meal, then you had better find six carbohydrate blocks to add to it and add another six external fat blocks. That could be two slices of bread and one apple with 1 tablespoon of mayonnaise. That's a pretty big sandwich, but when cut in half, it becomes two three-block meals. Or your choice may be a massive salad containing a head of lettuce, three tomatoes, two onions, and three green peppers, with six tablespoons of olive oil and vinegar dressing. Again, splitting this salad into two portions will also give you two three-block meals. And if that seems too much, then reduce the size of the salad and have a piece of fruit. The choice is yours, as long as you maintain your hormonal carburetor.

What about high-fat foods, such as peanuts? Most people think of peanuts as a high-protein food, because they are taught that peanut butter is a great source of protein for young kids. In reality, both peanuts and peanut butter are great sources of fat with a little protein and carbohydrate thrown in. Let's look at a typical label for peanuts.

First, I hope you are not going to eat the entire jar, since one serving of peanuts (unlike tuna fish) is about 1 ounce (fifteen individual nuts). In those fifteen nuts you are going to have 11 grams of fat, 6 grams of protein, and 7 grams of carbohydrate. Breaking this down to blocks would give nine fat blocks (11 grams divided by 1.5 grams equals nine blocks), one protein block (6 grams divided by 7 grams equals approximately one block), and one carbohydrate block (7 grams divided by 9 grams equals approximately one block). So while the peanuts (and other seeds and nuts) have an

Nutrition Facts

Serving Size 1oz.
Servings 16

Amount Per Serving

Calories 150   Calories from Fat 90

% Daily Value*

Total Fat 11g

    Saturated Fat 1.5g

Cholesterol 0mg

Sodium 115mg

Potassium 180mg

Total Carbohydrate 7g

    Dietary Fiber 2g

    Sugars 0g

Protein 6g

Figure 10-4. Label for Peanuts

appropriate protein-to-carbohydrate ratio, they are essentially all fat as far as the Zone is concerned. But they *can* be used to add extra fat to other meals that are too low in fat, to optimize your hormonal carburetor (and this is especially true of fresh-ground or natural peanut butter, which contains no additives, only ground peanuts).

Now that you are understanding how to break down food labels into blocks, let's take the next step and find a typical frozen dinner to see how it stacks up. Figure 10–5 shows the food labeling for a typical low-fat meal: Weight Watchers Ravioli Florentine.

Nutrition Facts

Serving Size 1
Servings 1

Amount Per Serving

Calories 220   Calories from Fat 15

% Daily Value*

Total Fat 2g

    Saturated Fat 0g

Cholesterol 5mg

Sodium 450mg

Potassium   mg

Total Carbohydrate 43g

    Dietary Fiber 4g

    Sugars 10g

Protein 9g

Figure 10-5. Label for Low-Fat Ravioli

The first thing you see is that the meal is low-fat (because you're still focusing on the fat content), with a total of 2 grams. In fact, the back of the box says, "How can it be so low in fat . . . and so delicious?" But 2 grams of fat is approximately one fat block (2 grams divided by 1.5 grams equals approximately one block). Now go to the carbohydrate content, and notice we have 43 grams. But bear in mind what is important is the insulin-promoting carbohydrate content. Since the meal has 4 grams of fiber, we should subtract this amount from the total of 43 grams of carbohydrate, leaving 39 grams of insulin-promoting carbohydrate. This translates into four carbohydrate blocks (39 grams divided by 9 grams equals approximately four blocks). So what about the protein? Well, it has only 9 grams of protein, which equals about one block of protein (9 grams divided by 7 grams is approximately one block). This ratio of four carbohydrate blocks to one protein block is just about the same as a Hershey's Chocolate Bar with Almonds—no wonder it's so delicious.

So before you eat this frozen dinner, how can you make it hormonally correct? First, it needs more protein. Since the frozen dinner contains four blocks of carbohydrate, we need to add another three blocks of protein to give it a total of four protein blocks. So go into your refrigerator and get 3 ounces of turkey breast or tuna fish to eat with this frozen dinner. But you're still not quite there. You need three more blocks of fat, and we are going to make this monounsaturated fat. The easiest way to do this is add three macadamia nuts or 3 teaspoons of slivered almonds. Now we have a hormonal winner, even though it started out as a hormonal loser. And the total calories with all these extra protein and fat additions? 365! The hormonal winner is also low-calorie. Not nearly as appetizing as the hundreds of Zone meals in Chapter 9, but at least it's a relatively fast meal that won't take you out of the Zone.

The best thing to do is to shop for fresh stuff and make it yourself. After all, who wants to eat frozen meals when they can enjoy family recipes handed down over the generations? People eat maybe ten favorite meals at home, because they tend to like the same meals over and over again. So why not take each of these ten favorite family meals and transform them into hormonal winners, just as we did for the Weight Watchers Ravioli Florentine, to be eaten and enjoyed again and again.

11

EATING OUT IN THE ZONE

Who actually eats in the Zone? Surprisingly, the French and Northern Italians come close without trying. These two cultures and cuisines are noted for being incredibly refined and sophisticated.

Think about the very posh four-star French restaurant. For fifty dollars you get a glass of great wine, a small amount of protein in the center of the plate, covered with a delicious sauce and surrounded by an artistically arranged outer ring of vegetables, and a small side salad to cleanse the palate. Even though you could have gobbled down five meals at the all-you-can-eat pasta palace for less than you paid at the four-star French restaurant, the French restaurant is serving you a Zone meal: adequate amounts of protein, low glycemic vegetables, and perhaps a glass of wine. And the four-star Northern Italian restaurant? For the same fifty dollars you now get a glass of wine, a piece of fish in the center of the plate, surrounded by an outer ring of artistically prepared vegetables, and a small side dish of pasta.

Neither of these meals was more than 500 calories (a Zone Diet rule), and each had an appropriate balance of protein to carbohydrate (another Zone Diet rule). And no one can accuse you of not having a great meal.

But how do you play the game when you're going out to a typical restaurant where a satisfied customer is one who has to unbuckle his belt after the meal? Here are some simple rules to follow at any restaurant, four-star or family style.

1. Rule #1. Never eat the rolls. If you're going to eat unfavorable carbohydrates, save them for dessert.

2. Rule #2. Always choose your low-fat protein entree from the menu first. This sets the stage for selecting the rest of your meal.

3. Rule #3. Always ask the waiter to replace the rice, potatoes, or pasta with vegetables. You will be amazed how gracious the restaurant will be.

4. Rule #4. While you're waiting for dinner, have a glass of red wine or a glass of bottled water while everyone else is munching on rolls. Try conversation instead of eating to pass the time.

5. Rule #5. Once the dinner is served, use the eyeball method to survey the scene. Look at the size of the low-fat protein entree you ordered. If it is significantly greater in size than the palm of your hand, plan to take the excess home (it sure beats eating cottage cheese the next day). Then look at your plate and determine whether the carbohydrates are favorable or unfavorable.

6. Rule #6. The volume of the low-fat protein you plan to eat determines the volume of the carbohydrate you are going to eat. If you're eating favorable carbohydrates, then you can have double the volume of carbohydrates compared to your protein portion. If you are planning to eat unfavorable carbohydrates, then you can eat only the same volume of carbohydrates as in your protein portion.

7. Rule #7. If you really came to the restaurant to eat dessert, then don't eat any carbohydrates (favorable or unfavorable) at your meal. When the server comes back with a dessert menu, order whatever you want, but plan to eat only half of it (remember, you have saved up your carbohydrate allotment, so now it's time to cash in). The rest of the dessert? Offer it to your dinner companions. I'm sure they will be delighted to help out. And the best dessert? Try fresh fruit.

Now that wasn't too difficult. It's very easy to do in the four-star restaurant, where there isn't very much food to begin with. It's much more difficult to undertake at the typical American restaurant in which great masses of food are shoved in your direction. This is what has happened to American restaurants in the last generation. Because we have the cheapest food on earth, people expect to get their money's worth by consuming massive amounts of calories. Everything is oversized (the only exceptions are the above-mentioned four-star restaurants where presentation and quality count for more than sheer bulk). And since mass is in, restaurant owners make their money by making sure most of the mass comes in the form of carbohydrates (which are dirt cheap) as opposed to protein (which is relatively expensive).

But it can be easy to order hormonally correct meals, even in fast-food restaurants, if you keep in mind the rules from the last chapter. Let's take McDonald's, for example. Here's a very quick Zone meal. Buy two inexpensive, small hamburgers, then throw one of the buns away. Put the two patties together in the remaining bun, and enjoy. A little high on the saturated fat and all unfavorable carbohydrates, but if you're not doing it very often, it's not too bad hormonally. Now here's a far better choice at McDonald's: buy the grilled McChicken sandwich and a salad. Throw away three-quarters of the bun, add the grilled chicken and the rest of the bun (as croutons) to the salad, and, presto, you have a grilled chicken salad with a touch of bread. It's quick, it's easy, and it's hormonally correct.

Fast-food restaurants can be a great help to you when you don't have the time to cook or to sit down at a restaurant. A more comprehensive summary of many of those fast-food meals can be found in *The Zone,* but the best quick meals can be found in your supermarket at the salad bar. Simply grab a bunch of precut vegetables and fruits (especially the things you would never buy otherwise) and put them in the aluminum plate they provide along with some olives (your monounsaturated fat). Then walk over to the deli and buy a quarter pound of low-fat protein, like turkey, chicken, or tuna. Add the low-fat protein to the precut vegetables, fruits, and olives, and you've got a great hormonal meal. It may be a little expensive compared to a bagel and a cup of coffee, but isn't your health worth it?

What if you're constantly on the road? How do you stay in the Zone? Here are some easy tricks for the business-trip road warrior. If you are going to be staying a couple of days at a hotel that has a room refrigerator, go out and buy some fruit and sliced low-fat deli meat or low-fat cottage cheese. For every 1/2 piece of fruit, plan to eat 1 ounce of low-fat deli meat or 2 ounces of cottage cheese. These can be quick snacks before you go out to eat (thereby making it easier to eat a Zone meal at the restaurant). And before you go to bed, remember to have a quick hormonal "touch-up" so that you get a good night's sleep in a strange bed.

Keep in mind that if you are a business person on the road, meals are your key to success because they are the main determinant of your mental alertness throughout the day. Here are three more hormonal winners you can always choose: For breakfast, have a three-egg omelette (try to have it made with egg substitutes or egg whites) and the fruit bowl, but don't eat the toast or the hash browns. For lunch, have a grilled chicken salad. And for dinner, eat fish with an extra serving of vegetables instead of the rice or potato. And, of course, never eat the rolls. Life is tough enough on the road without having to wander out of the Zone.

Eating out in the Zone is easy, if you know the rules. To quote Nancy Reagan, "just say no" to the overwhelming incoming tide of carbohydrates you're constantly exposed to when you eat. If you think it's difficult, then think of carbohydrates as a drug. The more you take of any drug, the more likely you are to get a drug overdose. In this case, an overdose of carbohydrates will generate an excess production of insulin, which can eventually kill you. That thought should make it easier to pass on the rolls the next time around.

12

YOUR ZONE REPORT CARD

The most important question a physician can ask a patient is "How do you feel?" That's the same question you want to ask yourself on the Zone Diet. My basic rule, whether it applies to a new diet, a vitamin, a mineral, an herb, etc., is to use as directed for two weeks. If you don't feel significantly better, then it's probably not going to happen.

The Zone Diet is no different. What results are you initially looking for? If you are like most people, you are after three simple things: thinking better, performing better, and looking better.

How do you think better? Once you begin to stabilize your blood sugar levels, you can expect your thinking to become much clearer and more focused. Think of what happens when you eat a big pasta meal at noon. By three o'clock you can barely keep your eyes open. The worst nightmare for a business executive is trying to negotiate a big business deal in the afternoon after eating a huge pasta lunch. If you want the world's greatest productivity tool, then think about following the Zone Diet.

Next, you should be performing better. When you're in the Zone, you essentially have a hormonal ATM card to tap into your body's stored fat, a virtually unlimited source of energy. So you should have more energy to spare for work, at home, and for play.

And finally, you will be looking better. You don't lose weight rapidly on a Zone Diet, but you do lose excess body fat at near a genetic maximum, which is 1 to 1½ pounds of fat per week. At the end of two weeks, your clothes, especially around your waist, will fit much better.

Even if you are having great success on the Zone Diet, every thirty days I strongly recommend that you eat a big carbohydrate-rich meal, like pasta. Why would you want to descend into carbohydrate hell? Just to let yourself know the difference between being in the Zone versus being out of it, even for one meal. What can you expect after eating that high-carbohydrate meal? An insulin hangover with loss of mental focus after the meal, grogginess and trouble waking the next morning, puffiness in your hands and feet, etc. It's a very instructive lesson on the hormonal power of food. Consider it a form of dietary Anabuse (Anabuse is a drug used to treat alcoholics that makes them violently ill when they drink any alcohol). Don't worry, however; you're only one meal away from getting right back into the Zone.

And what about meals? How do you know if you're making a hormonally winning meal? Well, you could do a radioimmune assay on your blood insulin levels every two hours, but that's pretty unrealistic. Or you could take blood sugar tests every two hours. Again, pretty unlikely. The easiest test is to just ask yourself how you feel during the next four to five hours after a meal. If you maintain a sharp mental focus and have no hunger for that four- to five-hour period, then you know the meal was a hormonal winner. Put that exact meal, with its ingredients and exact amounts, in your winner's cookbook so that you can come back to it at any time in the future. As with any drug, that meal will induce the same hormonal response.

Try to make your hormonal cookbook as large as possible. For most people that cookbook need consist of about only ten meals. Why? Well, most people really don't eat that many different meals at home. Of course, if you are like my wife and me, you probably have a million cookbooks as a result of joining some cookbook club years ago, but you still eat the same few meals you like to eat again and again. If each of those meals is a hormonal winner, eating any one of them will be the same as taking the most powerful drug known in order to think better, perform better, and look better. Most people would pay ungodly sums of money for such drugs, yet they exist right in your recipe file of hormonally winning meals.

Of course, feeling better, thinking better, performing better, and looking better are indicators that you're in the Zone, but in this age of technology most people want some hard numbers to confirm that they're feeling better. What can you do on your own to confirm that beneficial physiological changes are indeed happening? The first thing to track is the change in your percent body fat. You know your clothes are fitting better, but the weight on the scale isn't changing all that quickly. The reason you look at the scale at all is for a number that confirms the better fit of your clothes. Your weight, however, isn't nearly as important as your percent body fat in analyzing your overall health. So recalculate your percent body fat to confirm that your clothes are really fitting better. Using the tables in Appendix C allows you to make this measurement on a weekly basis.

And just how reliable are the tables found in the appendix? To answer that question, I did a study at the Medical Research Foundation in Houston, comparing the percent body fat of normal individuals determined by the tables in *The Zone* to the same number done by dual energy X-ray absorptiometry (DEXA) measurements (the new high-tech standard for measuring body fat). The variance of the results from the method in the appendix compared to the DEXA measurements was only about 1–2 percent in the body fat results. You might take a DEXA test once in your life, but you *can* measure yourself every day. Bear in mind that everything is relative to your starting point. And as you lower your percent body fat, know that you are lowering your insulin levels, too. As you lower your insulin levels, it is much more likely you are going to stay in the center of the Zone.

What if you still want more numbers? Well, this means getting a blood test. Most people (including me) hate seeing their blood leave their bodies. But when you know you're feeling better, you want every test in the book to confirm it. Most people dread going to a doctor's office to have a blood test, because they know they're there because they're sick, and they know the test is only going to confirm how sick they really are. Not surprisingly, when you're feeling great, you want to march in and demand as many tests as possible to congratulate yourself, if you only knew which tests.

One of the best is your blood pressure. No needles, no blood. It turns out that blood pressure is very sensitive to hyperinsulinemia. When you're done checking your blood pressure, have your physician take a blood sample (it's amazing how much braver you become in the Zone) and tell him or her you want the following tests:

- Fasting triglycerides
- HDL cholesterol
- Fasting-triglyceride-to-HDL-cholesterol ratio
- Fasting insulin
- Glycosylated hemoglobin (HgA$_1$C)

These are standard tests, but the last two are not routinely done, because they tend to be slightly more expensive. What results are you looking for? Your fasting triglycerides should be under 100 mg/dL, and your HDL cholesterol should be more than 50 mg/dL. This means your triglyceride-to-HDL-cholesterol ratio should be less than 2.0. Your fasting insulin should be less than 10 μ units/ml, and the HgA$_1$C should be less than 5 percent. The ratio of triglycerides to HDL cholesterol is indicative of your insulin levels. The higher the ratio, the higher your insulin. Likewise, your fasting insulin tells exactly how high your insulin levels are. Finally, the glycosylated hemoglobin tells you how well you have been keeping your blood sugar under control on a long-term basis. The lower your glycosylated hemoglobin, the better you have kept your insulin under control. The numbers of these clinical parameters give you very objective goals to mark your progress. In other words, your blood tells you whether you have been naughty or nice. These are your goals. It may take a little time to reach them, but if you are thinking better, performing better, and looking better as you progress toward them, you can afford the time.

Why are these numbers important? Because they indicate the extent of any hyperinsulinemia and therefore your likelihood of moving out of the Zone and toward chronic disease. If your triglycerides are greater than 200 mg/dL and your HDL cholesterol is less than 35 mg/dL, you're headed for big trouble, because you're hyperinsulinemic. Likewise, a fasting insulin greater than 15 μ units/ml means you're in danger, because you're hyperinsulinemic. And a glycosylated hemoglobin of greater than 9 percent means you're at high risk, because you're hyperinsulinemic.

Why do these numbers place you in such clinical trouble? It turns out that the primary risk factor that determines your likelihood to develop heart disease is not high cholesterol levels, or high blood pressure, but elevated insulin levels. If you're hyperinsulinemic, you'll be making more of a certain group of hormones (i.e., "bad" eicosanoids) that can actually make you ill. And if you have read *The Zone*, you know that represents very big trouble.

Why doesn't medical science just find some drug that lowers insulin? Actually, such a drug exists: It's called food. If you're hyper-insulinemic, then start using that drug. Your life depends on it.

13

LIVING IN THE ZONE

There's more to living in the Zone than simply eating. You really
want to do everything you can to keep your insulin levels from
rising.

What you eat and how you eat will have the greatest impact on
getting you to the Zone, but there are two other ways you can
enhance your diet to get to the Zone and stay there on a permanent
basis. Not surprisingly, just like eating, you can do these things
yourself. These extra magical hormonal elixirs are exercise and
stress reduction. Before you go off to join some gym or find an
appropriate guru in India, let me give you some very simple ways
to integrate these two hormonal control strategies into your everyday life.

EXERCISE—JUST DO IT

The very word inspires dread for most people. Not because you
don't think it's important, you just don't have the time to do it. There
are two types of exercise you should do every day: aerobic and
anaerobic.

Aerobic exercise simply means doing exercise that requires oxygen. As I pointed out in *The Zone,* the best exercise for most people is walking. Simply walk fifteen minutes in one direction, then
turn around and walk back. You can do this in the morning, at
lunch, after dinner. Just plan to do it once a day. You can even park
your car a fifteen-minute walk from work, walk to your job, and
then walk back to your car after work.

You don't need to join a health club, buy a designer Spandex
exercise outfit, or invest in a pair of high-tech running shoes. That

isn't to say there aren't benefits to more intensive aerobic exercise, but make this daily walking an integral part of your life before you decide to increase your level of activity. I have for one never yet figured out the logic of having valet parking at posh health clubs in California. Why not just park the car down the street and walk to the club?

What about anaerobic exercise, isn't that weightlifting? And doesn't this mean joining some dark and dingy gym surrounded by hulking figures that come out of central casting? No, in fact all the weight training you'll probably ever need can be done in your bedroom or for that matter any hotel room if you are on the road. All it takes is about five minutes a day.

The weight you're going to use is your own body, and you carry that piece of equipment with you wherever you go. You should work your upper and lower body muscles at every workout and you can do it with two simple exercises: pushups and squats.

Let's start with pushups. Many people, especially women, will have trouble doing a pushup at first, especially if they're out of shape. The key to all upper body exercises is to always keep your back straight. Correct form is always more important than the number of repetitions.

If you are really in bad shape, initially just lean toward a wall and push yourself away. These are really push-aways, not pushups. When you can easily do three sets of about ten to fifteen of these push-aways, then you're ready to progress to the next level, which is counter-pushes. Stand two to three feet away from a counter. With your hands on the counter, lower your body toward it and then push yourself away. After you can do three sets of ten to fifteen of these counter-pushes, you're ready for knee pushups (you're getting closer to that "dreaded" pushup all the time). Now simply kneel on the floor with your chest touching the floor. Place your hands on the floor at shoulder width and push your upper body up, keeping your knees touching the floor. After you can easily do three sets of knee pushups ten to fifteen times, you're finally ready for the traditional pushup. These are just like the knee pushups except now you lift your knees off the floor along with your upper body. All of your weight now rests upon your hands and your toes. Lower yourself until you are about one inch from the ground, and then raise yourself back up. Your goal is to do three sets of ten to fifteen of these traditional pushups on a daily basis.

Pushups are great for the upper body, but what about the lower body? For that you want to do squats (also described by your grandmother as deep knee bends). Squats are deceptive, because they require a lot of lower body strength. As with pushups, it's always best to start slowly, and always keep your back straight. Begin by using a chair with arms. Sit down and then stand up. If you initially have to use the arms of the chair for support, that's OK. Do three sets of this ten to fifteen times in each set. Your next progression is to do the same exercise without using the arms of the chair for support. The next step is to cross your arms across your chest and still be able to do three sets of ten to fifteen repetitions. Once you can do that, you're in position to begin to do a squat, which is essentially sitting down on a chair that isn't there. Don't let your knees bend more than 90 degrees, and at first do these squats with your arms extended. Once you reach that goal of three sets of ten to fifteen repetitions, then do the same exercise with your arms crossed on your chest.

So here's your daily exercise routine. Do one set of pushups (at whatever level you can), followed by one set of squats (at whatever level you can). Rest one minute, and then repeat both exercises again. Rest another minute and do both the pushups and squats a third time. When you can easily do fifteen repetitions on the third and last set, then go to the next level of difficulty the following day. The total time of your anaerobic exercise is five minutes a day in the privacy of your own home or in a hotel room if you're traveling. Just do it every day.

If you're walking thirty minutes a day and doing five minutes a day of strength training, you've got a pretty good exercise program. And you would be surprised how many people will still complain about the time it takes to do even this level of exercise. But if you really want to get into the Zone, this small expenditure of time and effort is certainly worth it.

Even if you have reached this level of exercise, before you join a health club, I would first recommend that you just buy a set of light barbells weighing between 1 and 15 pounds (or fill old plastic milk bottles that have handles partially with water, then grasp them by the handles) to do strength exercises in addition to your standard pushups and squats. Your pushups and squats now become great warm-ups for additional weight-bearing exercises. Any number of exercise books will describe more advanced barbell exercises for both the lower and upper body. The key point is that you should never let more than one minute go by between sets and should try not to go more than thirty minutes of exercise with weights. Beyond that point, hormonal levels begin to change significantly (i.e., testosterone drops and cortisol rises), and you can gain very little additional benefit with increased training. And if you want more aerobic activity? Walk one hour per day.

STRESS REDUCTION—STOP AND SMELL THE ROSES

Stress is a biochemical event that causes significant hormonal responses. The acute stress brought on by danger causes the release of hormones, such as adrenaline, which mobilize you for the typical "flight or fight" syndrome associated with acute stress. However, what is more common in our present society is chronic stress, which also has other hormonal consequences. During chronic stress, the hormone cortisol is being released at an elevated level. As cortisol levels rise, insulin resistance increases, which in turn causes insulin levels to rise. It's these rising insulin levels that drive you out of the Zone. The so-called Type A personality (aggressive, hard-charging, driven, etc.) is the type of individual with increased cortisol levels. And since cardiovascular disease is associated with such Type A personalities, it is not surprising that stress reduction can play an important role in reducing heart attack.

You don't have to find a guru or chant mantras all day long to reduce stress. Just carve out some personal time for the things you like to do (and I hope watching TV is not one of them). Probably the best stress reducer is walking. Not power walks where you are trying to pump up your heart rate, but the type of walks that let you stop and talk to neighbors, or enjoy the scenery, or even smell the roses. In each of these cases, there is a lot of stopping and starting, but since you have no particular agenda, it's a great stress reducer. Furthermore, walking is a two-in-one activity. Besides reducing stress, you're also reducing insulin by exercising aerobically. And insulin reduction is what it's all about.

So there you have it—diet, exercise, and stress reduction. Three low-tech ways to treat a high-tech problem: hyperinsulinemia. These are things you can begin tomorrow as you start your journey toward the Zone. Not only will these steps get you to the Zone, but they will allow you to live regularly there.

DRUGS THAT TAKE YOU OUT OF THE ZONE

You should be aware that a number of drugs can take you out of the Zone by raising insulin levels. Two of the most common are diuretics and beta-blockers, both commonly used in the treatment of high blood pressure. Newer hypertensive drugs such as angiotensin-converting enzyme (ACE) inhibitors have no effect on insulin levels. Corticosteroids, such as prednisone, also significantly raise insulin levels. Then there is another drug that only slightly elevates insulin levels. Unfortunately, that drug is ubiquitous in America. It's called caffeine. And one of the best ways to help yourself get to the Zone is to reduce the use of that drug.

14

FREQUENTLY ASKED QUESTIONS ABOUT THE ZONE

GENERAL

If I follow the Zone Diet, does this mean I can never have rice, pasta, and bagels again?

Of course not. Following a Zone Diet only means that you should be using these sources of carbohydrates in moderation, like condiments. Simply make sure that most of your daily intake of carbohydrates comes from fruits and vegetables.

Do I have to be obsessive about the Zone Diet to be successful?

No. Obviously, the greater the precision, the greater the results, but if you only play by the rules of the Zone Game and use the eyeball method, you won't be too far away from the center of the Zone. Just remember to pay very close attention to your responses after a meal. Using the simple tools in this book, you will be able to adjust your hormonal carburetor with increasing precision without having to obsess about portion size, blocks, and calculations.

Should I be concerned about such a seemingly low daily caloric intake?

If you have excess body fat (greater than 15 percent for males and greater than 22 percent for females), then all the calories you need are already stored in your body. Remember that the typical male or female in this country carries about 100,000 calories of stored fat at all times. To put this in perspective, this represents approximately 1,700 pancakes, which is a pretty big breakfast. To access those 1,700 pancakes you simply need a "hormonal ATM card" to release these stored calories. The Zone Diet is that card. If you are using that ATM card correctly, you don't have to consume as many external calories to meet your body's energy requirements. On the Zone Diet, you are eating *as if* you are already at your ideal percentage of body fat because you are using a combination of your stored body fat and incoming calories to meet your total caloric requirements.

Doesn't any low-calorie diet cause fat loss?

Not necessarily. Research studies in the 1950s conducted by Kekwick and Pawan at the Middlesex Hospital in London examined diets consisting of 1,000 calories per day. All patients lost substantial weight on a high-protein (90 percent of calories) diet, high-fat (90 percent of calories) diet, and mixed (42 percent of calories as carbohydrate) diets, but most patients actually gained weight on a high-carbohydrate (90 percent of calories) diet. Cutting back on calories without gaining access to your hormonal ATM card is a surefire prescription for deprivation, constant hunger, and fatigue. Any time you reduce calories, you will lose some weight, but eventually you hit a hormonal plateau where the weight loss (and more importantly, fat loss) stops, but feelings of hunger, deprivation, and fatigue continue. The Zone Diet is not a diet; it's a hormonal control program that allows you to optimize your quality of life.

What is more important, the amount of carbohydrates you consume or the glycemic index of the carbohydrates you eat?

The total intake of carbohydrates is most important. However, you will get even greater results on the Zone Diet by making sure most of your carbohydrates come from low-glycemic carbohydrates. By eating low-glycemic foods, you are retarding their rates of entry into the bloodstream, thereby maintaining the best possible balance of your insulin levels. In addition, low-glycemic carbohydrates provide the maximum amounts of vitamins and minerals with the least amount of carbohydrate. Finally, by eating primarily low-glycemic carbohydrates, you will constantly be faced with a very hearty meal because low-glycemic carbohydrates are also usually low-density carbohydrates. It is simply very hard, if not impossible, to overconsume low-density carbohydrates such as fruits and vegetables.

How long before I can expect to see results on the Zone Diet?

Within two to three days you should see a noticeable reduction in your carbohydrate cravings and increased mental focus. Within five days you will notice a significant increase in your lack of hunger throughout the day, coupled with better physical performance. Within two weeks, although you will not have lost much weight, you will notice that your clothes are fitting much better. Keep in mind the maximum fat loss you can expect is 1 to 1½ pounds of fat per week. It is simply impossible to reduce excess body fat any faster.

Why doesn't the Zone Diet include the protein content of carbohydrate-rich sources like vegetables or grains?

Because people would get too bogged down in the calculations. A significant amount of the protein in these foods is not absorbed; therefore one has to impose correction factors to take into account the actual amount of protein that is absorbed and thus its effect on hormonal response. Since vegetable sources are not very protein-dense, it makes more sense to ignore their protein contribution. Vegetarians should make sure that they always include protein-rich vegetarian sources such as firm tofu, isolated protein powders, or soybean imitation meat products at every meal to ensure adequate protein intake.

What is the minimum amount of daily protein block intake?

Regardless of your protein calculations, we always recommend a minimum of eight protein blocks throughout the day for adults.

Won't a high-protein diet cause osteoporosis and kidney failure?

Not if you are eating a protein-adequate diet like the Zone Diet. No one should be eating more protein than his or her body requires, but, conversely, no one should be eating less, because to do so is to put yourself in a state of protein malnutrition. On the Zone Diet, not only are you eating adequate protein, but you are spreading it over three meals and two snacks. It's almost as if you are receiving an intravenous drip of protein. Excessive protein at any meal can't be stored by the body, and therefore has to be converted into fat. The first step in this conversion process is the removal of the amino group from the protein, which can put a strain on the kidneys if excessive protein is floating around in the bloodstream. Furthermore, the newest research indicates that even for patients with kidney failure, the earlier reports about the benefits of protein restriction may have been overstated. The calcium loss often associated with eating excessive amounts of protein is completely blocked if adequate dietary calcium is supplied with the protein. The one mineral many women don't get enough of is calcium. So if you are concerned, drink a glass of milk with each meal or take a calcium supplement.

Why don't the French have high rates of heart disease?

Nutritionists just hate the French. They smoke, they drink, they eat lots of fat, they don't exercise, they seem to have a very good time, and they have the lowest rates of heart disease in Europe. It's called the French Paradox. It's only a paradox if it is contrary to your expectations. Obviously, there are a number of reasons for these surprising statistics, but I believe the major factor is that their meals are moderate in calories, are rich in fruits and vegetables, always contain protein, and include fat. That's basically the Zone Diet. We also have the so-called Spanish Paradox. In the last twenty years, Spaniards have eaten more protein, more fat, and fewer grains than they used to as a population and their rates of cardiovascular disease are dropping. These are not paradoxes, simply adjustments in the hormonal responses of a population to a changing diet.

The Chinese eat a lot of rice; don't they have low rates of heart disease?

No, according to the American Heart Association. The rates of cardiovascular disease in urban Chinese males are nearly as great as the rates for Americans, and Chinese females, both rural and urban, actually have greater rates of cardiovascular disease than American females.

I'm concerned about pesticides on fruits and vegetables, and the hormones and antibiotics used in beef and chicken production. What should I do?

These are valid concerns. You should always try to eat organic fruits and vegetables and range-fed beef and chicken. However, be prepared to pay a significantly higher price and be willing to cope with reduced availability. Don't, however, make this an excuse for not eating the appropriate protein-to-carbohydrate ratio at every meal.

I'm not overweight. Why would I need to follow the Zone Diet?

The Zone Diet is not a diet. It's a lifelong hormonal control program. Loss of excess body fat is only a side effect (although a very beneficial side effect). The Zone Diet was originally developed for cardiovascular patients, and was tested on world-class athletes. Between those two extremes lies everyone else. If you are at your ideal percent body fat, and want to think better and perform better, then the Zone Diet is for you.

When was the Zone Diet developed?

The program has been undergoing constant testing and revision since 1984. The present program represents the seventh generation of my original concept to control hormonal responses using dietary intervention. *The Zone* provides a more detailed history of this development process. The Zone Diet has been used by thousands of individuals during this developmental period since 1984.

Can I still continue to use my vitamins and minerals?

Vitamins and minerals are an excellent low-cost insurance policy to ensure adequate levels of micronutrients. However, a Zone Diet—which is primarily composed of low-fat protein, fruits, and vegetables—provides an excellent base of vitamins and minerals, and requires much less supplementation. The only supplement that I strongly recommend is extra vitamin E, since the Zone Diet is still a low total fat diet, and most dietary vitamin E comes from fat.

What exactly do you mean by "use in moderation" when referring to unfavorable carbohydrates?

Try not to make unfavorable carbohydrates (grains, starches, breads, and pasta) more than 25 percent of the total carbohydrate blocks in a meal. Use them as condiments, not the primary source of your carbohydrate intake.

Should I be concerned about sodium?

Not if you are following a Zone Diet, because excess insulin activates another hormonal system that promotes sodium retention. However, it always makes sense not to use excessive amounts of sodium.

I'm a pure vegetarian. How can I make this diet work for me?

Simply add protein-rich vegetarian foods to your existing diet to maintain the correct protein-to-carbohydrate ratio. Ideal choices would be firm and extra-firm tofu and isolated soybean protein powder. The new generation of soybean-based imitation meat products (hot dogs, hamburgers, sausages, etc.) are another excellent way of getting protein-rich vegetarian foods into your existing meals. Traditional vegetarian protein sources, such as beans, have an exceptionally high amount of carbohydrate for the amount of protein they provide, which makes it impossible to achieve the desired protein-to-carbohydrate ratio needed to enter the Zone.

Which protein powders are best?

Excellent sources of isolated protein include egg and milk combinations and lactose-free whey powder. For vegetarians, isolated soy protein powders are excellent choices. Protein powders are available at most health food stores. These protein powders can be added to carbohydrate-rich meals, like oatmeal, to make them more hormonally favorable. They can also be added to flours and mixes (such as pancake, muffin, and cookie mixes) for cooking and baking to fortify the protein content.

What impact will various cooking methods have on the quality of the macronutrients or micronutrients?

Cooking has little effect on the macronutrients (except that excessive heat can damage and cross-link protein with carbohydrates). However, cooking can have a significant negative effect on micronutrients (vitamins and minerals). Vitamins are extraordinarily sensitive to heat. And minerals can be leached out of food when cooked with water. Therefore, steaming vegetables is an ideal preparation method to retain micronutrients and yet make the vegetables more digestible. Fruits are usually eaten raw, retaining all their micronutrients. The more carbohydrates are processed or cooked, the more rapid their rate of entry into the bloodstream. This is why instant forms of carbohydrate like instant rice or instant potatoes should be avoided.

Do I eat my meal or snack even if I'm not hungry?

Yes. This is the best time to eat in order to maintain hormonal equilibrium from one meal to the next.

Will this diet heal the damage done to my body over the years?

The body has a remarkable ability to repair itself, given the appropriate tools. The best of those tools is the diet, especially one that orchestrates the appropriate hormonal responses that accelerate the repair process.

Why don't I count all the protein, carbohydrate, and fat in everything I eat?

Because you would probably need a mini-computer to make all the calculations. This is why we devised the block method that takes into account fat content and protein digestibility, the fat content in low-fat protein, and the insulin-sensitive carbohydrate content of carbohydrates, making your calculations for preparing each meal exceptionally simple.

Will a liquid meal in the correct ratio get me to the Zone? If not, why not?

A liquid meal has a much greater surface area than a solid food. As a result, the digestion and entry rate of macronutrients into the bloodstream cannot be controlled as well, and there is a corresponding decrease in the desired hormonal control. Liquid meals are more convenient, but they are not as hormonally desirable as solid food. They can be used occasionally if you just don't have the time to cook.

Can children use the Zone Diet?

The diet is ideal for children because they need to be in the Zone even more than adults. For children, assume that they have 10 percent body fat when you make their lean body mass calculations. Then, whatever their activity factor actually is, increase it by two levels. This is to ensure more than adequate protein for growth spurts. The one protein source that virtually every child will eat is string cheese. Although a little high in saturated fat, string cheese is a good way to begin to introduce more protein in your child's diet. That leaves just the hard part for parents: getting your kids to eat fruits and vegetables instead of pasta and bread.

How do I know that two years from now the Zone Diet will not turn out to be like the other diets that initially produce great results?

The Zone Diet is not a diet, but a lifelong hormonal control program that allows you to maximize your full genetic potential. These hormonal systems have evolved over the last forty million years and are unlikely to change soon. Surprisingly, many diets are based on gluttony. Eat either all the carbohydrate you want (high-carbohydrate, low-fat diets) or all the protein and fat you want (high protein, low-carbohydrate diets). The Zone Diet is based on moderation. There are limits on the amount of protein, carbohydrate, and fat consumed at every meal.

I'm off the body fat calculation charts found in **The Zone.** *What should I do?*

Assume that you have 50 percent body fat. With time you will lose sufficient fat so that you can follow the percent body fat charts. If you are off the weight charts, then also increase your physical activity level by one level, because with all the extra fat you have, you are essentially doing light weight training twenty-four hours a day.

FAT FACTS

Why do I need extra fat? What does it do?

Paradoxically it takes fat to burn fat, if that fat is monounsaturated fat. Remember, this is not an excuse for fat gluttony, but the need to add back reasonable amounts of fat to each meal. First, fat acts as a control rod to slow the rate of entry of carbohydrate into the bloodstream, thereby reducing the insulin response. Second, it releases a hormone (cholecystokinin, or CCK) from the stomach that tells the brain to stop eating. Third, it supplies the building blocks (i.e., essential fatty acids) for eicosanoids. Most of your fat intake should be in the form of monounsaturated fat, and the amount of fat you consume is dictated by the amount of protein you consume at each meal.

Can I lose too much body fat?

Obviously it's possible to lose too much body fat. So once you reach a percent of body fat that you are happy with and wish to stabilize your weight at that point, simply add more monounsaturated fat to your diet. This extra monounsaturated fat will act as a caloric ballast to provide the extra calories to maintain your percent body fat without affecting insulin levels. Why? Monounsaturated fat has no effect on insulin. It's hormonally neutral.

Why is a fat block only 1.5 grams?

Every block of low-fat protein contains approximately 1.5 grams of "hidden" fat. Therefore, by adding one extra fat block (which is defined as 1.5 grams of fat) for each block of low-fat protein, you are actually consuming 3 grams of fat or two fat blocks (one internal in the protein and one external) for each protein block. If you are using fat-free protein sources, such as isolated protein powders, then you should be adding two blocks of fat to achieve the same ratio. Obviously, if you are eating higher-fat protein choices, you would not be adding any extra fat blocks to your meal. Remember that every time you add additional fat blocks to a meal, they should be composed primarily of monounsaturated fat.

What's wrong with supplementing my diet with flaxseed oil?

A central theme in *The Zone* is the reduction of arachidonic acid levels by diet. Controlling insulin is your most powerful tool, but the addition of omega–3 fatty acids can also have a significant benefit. Flaxseed oil is rich in alpha linolenic acid (ALA), which is an omega–3 fatty acid and therefore has some use in controlling arachidonic acid production. But if you are going to supplement with an omega–3 oil, then I recommend fish oil, which is rich in the best omega–3 fatty acid, eicosapentaenoic acid (EPA). EPA has a tenfold greater impact on reducing the production of bad eicosanoids than does ALA on a gram-for-gram basis. Another reason I prefer fish oil over flaxseed oil is that the excess consumption of ALA in flaxseed oil tends to reduce the production of gamma linolenic acid (GLA), the building block of good eicosanoids. What's excess? Anything more than one tablespoon per day. Finally, the vast body of research data on the clinical benefits of EPA is overwhelming. Therefore, supplementation with EPA as opposed to ALA will have a far greater impact in getting you into the Zone. But before you add any omega–3 fatty acid supplements to your diet, try to get those fatty acids from food itself. The best source of EPA? Salmon. Of course, you could do what your grandmother did in her day to ensure adequate levels of EPA, and take cod liver oil.

Besides salmon, where can I get EPA, and how often should I eat fish each week?

Other sources that are rich in EPA include mackerel and sardines. Other marine sources that have a lower EPA content are common fish such as tuna, swordfish, scallops, shrimp, and lobster. Try to consume about 300 mg of EPA per week. This would translate into one serving of salmon or four servings of tuna or similar fish per week. One teaspoon of cod liver oil contains about 500 mg of EPA.

How can I tell if fish oil is safe?

The best indication that a fish oil capsule or cod liver oil containing EPA has been molecularly distilled, which removes harmful chemicals, is that it is cholesterol-free. This is a very expensive process that literally distills over chemicals, leaving the sensitive fish oil intact. This means that any residual PCBs, which contaminate virtually all fish and might be found in even refined fish oil, have been removed.

I'm a vegetarian and can't use fish oil. What should I do?

This is the one case I would suggest supplementation to your diet with flaxseed oil as a source of omega–3 fatty acids. But I would recommend no more than one tablespoon of refined flaxseed oil per day so that the natural production of GLA is not compromised.

FINE-TUNING

How do I adjust my hormonal carburetor?

Not everyone is genetically the same. Your hormonal carburetor is based on the protein-to-carbohydrate ratio that generates the best hormonal response for you. That hormonal response is easily measured by asking yourself, "How do I feel?" four to five hours after a meal. If you maintain excellent mental clarity and have no hunger, then the protein-to-carbohydrate ratio in the last meal you ate is correct for you. Your goal is to make every meal with that same ratio to generate the same hormonal response. For the vast majority of people, this ratio is 3 grams of protein for every 4 grams of effective carbohydrate. So the most efficient way to fine-tune your own carburetor is to start with this ratio and then experiment slightly on either side to determine your limits by using hunger and mental clarity as the parameters to optimize.

I'm still hungry on the Zone Diet. What should I do?

You need to make a slight adjustment to your hormonal carburetor. Always look back to your last meal. If you feel hungry within two to three hours after you eat, and experience a drop-off in mental focus (because of low blood sugar), it is because you consumed too much carbohydrate relative to the amount of protein. As a result, you're making too many bad eicosanoids because of an increase in insulin secretion that has taken you out of the Zone. Simply make that same meal in the future and keep the protein constant, but reduce the carbohydrate amount by one block. On the other hand, if you feel hungry before any four- to six-hour cycle ends, but maintain good mental focus, you're actually making too many good eicosanoids, which is pushing insulin levels too low. The brain has a sensing system that picks up low insulin levels in the bloodstream and tells you to eat to increase insulin levels, even though the brain is getting plenty of blood sugar (hence the good mental focus). Simply make that same meal in the future, and add one additional block of carbohydrate to the meal. In essence what you are doing is adjusting your personal hormonal carburetor to get to the center of the Zone. In either case, you should add more monounsaturated fat to either meal, as fat releases the hormone cholecystokinin (CCK), which promotes a feeling of fullness that is known as satiety.

I have developed some constipation. What should I do?

A Zone Diet will switch your body to a fat-burning metabolism instead of a carbohydrate-burning metabolism. The metabolism of fat requires greater amounts of water on a daily basis. So the first step is to increase your water intake by 50 percent. If this isn't sufficient to reduce the constipation, then it means that you are probably releasing stored arachidonic acid from your fat cells. For about 25 percent of the population, there will be a transitory release of stored arachidonic acid, the building block of bad eicosanoids, from stored body fat. The buildup of extra arachidonic acid in your stored fat is a result of your previous dietary patterns. This temporary increase in arachidonic acid can give rise to constipation by reducing water flow into the colon. Adding extra EPA to your diet will minimize this transitory effect. The best source of EPA is fish, but another good source is fish oil capsules. I would also recommend taking some crystalline vitamin C with each meal. Alternatively, you can slow down the access to your stored body fat by making a slight adjustment in your hormonal carburetor and adding one extra carbohydrate block to each meal.

As I drop weight, should I drop the number of protein blocks I eat?

No. The weight you are dropping is pure fat. The program is designed to maintain your lean body mass (LBM), which requires protein to maintain it. In essence, on the Zone Diet you are eating *as if* you are at your ideal body weight. The only time to change your protein block intake is when you change your physical activity level or see a significant change in your LBM, which you can measure using the tables found in *The Zone*. However, if you are overweight, you should recalculate your LBM after two weeks on the diet, since you may lose some retained water (which artificially inflates your real LBM, and therefore inflates your real protein requirements). This recalculation will provide you with your real LBM upon which to base your protein requirements.

Should I add protein if I'm trying to gain lean body mass? If so, how much?

The only way to build muscle mass is by exercise, primarily weight training. However, building one pound of new muscle mass per month is a noble goal. To do so, however, requires only one extra protein block per day in addition to the number of protein blocks required to maintain your existing lean body mass. One pound of new muscle equals 454 grams. But muscle is 70 percent water, which means that one pound of new muscle contains about 136 grams of protein. Divide 136 grams by 30 days, and you get 4.5 grams of extra protein per day required to build new muscle. Taking in one extra block of protein (7 grams) per day will be more than adequate in your quest to add one extra pound of muscle per month.

How should I alter this diet if I'm pregnant and/or nursing my child?

If you are pregnant or nursing, you should be using a Zone Diet to ensure adequate protein intake. For pregnant women, whatever your physical activity level actually is, increase it by two levels. For example, if you have a physical activity level of 0.7 grams of protein per pound of lean body mass, then increase it to 0.9 grams of protein per pound of lean body mass. For nursing mothers, increase your physical activity factor by one level over your actual physical activity level. However, if pregnant, always check with your physician before making any dietary change.

Can I cut back on fat blocks as long as I match my protein and carbohydrate requirements?

You can, but ironically you will not lose as much fat. The small amount of added fat acts as a control rod to reduce the rate of entry of carbohydrates into the bloodstream, thereby reducing insulin secretion. By reducing insulin, you can access your stored body fat more effectively. Also, the fat causes the release of the hormone cholecystokinin (CCK) that promotes satiety between meals. Of course, any added fat to your diet should be primarily monounsaturated fat, such as olive oil, guacamole, almonds, or macadamia nuts.

How do I get even more information?

Visit my site on the World Wide Web at http://www.Eicotech.com. This Web site is a virtual on-line Zone magazine, with weekly updates on new recipes, medical research news, and additional helpful tips to stay in the Zone. Consider this Web site your on-line Zone Community Center.

15

TALES FROM THE ZONE

Being in the Zone will help you think better, perform better, and look better. But the power of this dietary technology goes far beyond these benefits alone. It was developed to treat what I call "either/or" medical conditions: medical conditions that either have no treatment or those for which the treatments are less than desirable.

Hormonal control will be the key to twenty-first-century medicine, and much of this hormonal control comes from the food you eat: You take advantage of this fact when you enter the Zone. Once you are in the Zone, you are in position to control the most powerful hormones in your body, eicosanoids. You make over one hundred different types of these hormones, and they affect every cell in your body. They can keep you well or they can make you sick. You control them by controlling insulin levels. And you control insulin levels by your diet. The end result is that some very remarkable changes are possible if you treat food with the same respect that you treat a prescription drug.

While I can tell you this over and over, perhaps you would like to hear what other people have to say about the Zone Diet and how it has affected their life. These are their stories. They may begin like yours, or like the story of someone you know. Their endings, however, come straight from the Zone.

It's usually when you get bad news from your doctor that you begin to really appreciate health. And no news is worse than that your key organs are failing. Nothing can be more frightening than an organ transplant. The only time you undergo one is when you are literally days from death. Consider the story of Mary P., whose lung capacity was so compromised that she required a double lung transplant just to survive. Last year she began following the Zone Diet, and she won a gold medal in the 20-kilometer cycling event at the 1995 World Transplant Games. Nowadays, she routinely rides in 100-mile-plus events at the age of forty-nine. Does being in the Zone help? Mary likes to think so.

If organ transplants mean you're close to death, then having cancer is not far behind. Consider the tale of Willard H., a prostate cancer survivor who wrote,

I just returned from the Mayo Clinic where I go for my annual physical. All of my tests came out well. My PSA [a marker for prostate cancer] is undetectable. My cholesterol has continued to decrease from 210 to 150. Thanks and congratulations go to you and The Zone. I spoke with my physicians about the Zone Diet. They were not experts on nutrition, but said they thought it was a good program. Neither their encouragement nor discouragement would have made a difference with me. I'm on your program for life. I give a lot of credit to your program for keeping my PSA at the bottom end of the scale.

Reaching the Zone is all about this improved quality of life. That's why I particularly like the letter that I got from Joan S., who wrote:

This "incurable" multiple sclerosis is reversing after sixteen years. It feels like I'm living a miracle. I'm glad I've kept daily notes because it seems unbelievable. I keep pinching myself.

What is even more encouraging are letters from individuals who have been on medication for decades, like Louise P., who wrote the following:

For 40 years I have been taking thyroid pills and drugs against depression. In addition, I had high blood pressure of 180/95 that was only controlled by medication. Since my understanding of your concept pertaining to the Zone and applying its principles, I am a healthy person taking no more thyroid pills, no more anti-depressants, no more high blood pressure medications since my blood pressure is now 120/70. I thank you with the deepest gratitude for restoring my health through your dietary guidelines. And my husband and children feel the same way.

Reductions in blood pressure are common, as Steve W. wrote:

I tried your program and am very satisfied. My blood pressure was 132/103. Even after cutting out desserts and having my weight drop to 172, my blood pressure had not changed. After 45 days on the Zone Diet, my weight is in the low 160s but my blood pressure has dropped to 103/73. I guess you can say you probably saved my life. I am sorry I had to give up so many of my favorite things, such as bread, pizza, and rice. But I am developing new favorites such as cherries, peaches, blueberries, turkey breast and more. I guess it's a small price to pay to live longer.

I also received a letter from Pat G., who wrote:

I weighed 205 pounds and was a Type II diabetic. My brain was always foggy from the use of my medications. After 4 months on the Zone Diet, I have lost 41 pounds, I feel great. My body is still changing. My muscles are building and becoming more toned while I am losing fat. I take no medications. My blood sugar levels continue to remain in the normal range. I have very little, if any, pain now from my back and my leg. My doctor can't believe it.

Pat's experience in the Zone, with the resulting control of blood sugar, is no different from that of lots of other people, including Elisa L., who wrote:

During the month of September, I developed a strange taste of sawdust in my mouth and some needle pain in my liver, in addition to a small amount of foam in my urine. I decided to go to my doctor, and my blood tests of October 13 showed a fasting blood glucose level of 288, and inflammation of the liver. He prescribed a medication for diabetes, and then come back in 6 weeks for another test. I seriously pondered whether to try your Zone Diet and not the medication. I reported it to my doctor who, as expected, was not at all pleased. I bargained with him for four weeks of a trial. I confessed to him that I had abused my body for the last 40 years (I'm now 71), [and] therefore [wanted] to give my body a chance for recovery. Scared to death, I followed the Zone Diet to the letter. Four weeks later, my blood glucose test was 103, totally normal. Then, on purpose, I exited the Zone Diet a bit, and a week later my blood sugar had risen to 126. I am truly feeling that food must be perceived as a drug.

Relief from pain is crucial for quality of life. That's why I was happy to receive a letter from Belinda D. Belinda is a heath care professional who was not only overweight, but also suffered from repetitive stress injuries that had required three separate surgeries. She was still taking eighteen aspirins per day to ease the pain. In her letter, Belinda wrote:

When I picked up your book in the bookstore, my first response was to put it back on the shelf and renew my promise not to try a diet program. What made me stop and buy the book was the section I read on chronic pain and arthritis. At that point, I was ready to try anything. Within a month of following the Zone Diet, my pain levels were reduced to a point where I stopped taking all medication, and I was actually returning to basically pain-free living. The weight loss I have experienced has been an added bonus to the way I feel. For the record I have lost 40 pounds in the last five months. I have a ways to go, but I feel no stress in getting to my ideal weight. My husband has been equally as successful in the Zone. He has returned to his ideal weight of 178 (from 220), and it is like having a new man around the house. The biggest improvement has come in his emotional well-being. Thank you again for your work and for publishing the information in such a clear and concise manner.

There are many more stories like these, but I feel the examples I have chosen are representative of my basic premise that food is a very powerful drug if used correctly.

But what about overweight individuals who use exercise to lose weight? Consider Steve G., who three years ago weighed 313 pounds. Determined to change his life Steve started biking and running 1.5 hours per day and sticking to a 1,000-calorie diet rich in carbohydrates and low in fat. Within a year, he had reached 250. For the next year and a half, he did the same exercise and low-calorie, high-carbohydrate diet, and nothing happened. His weight remained the same. As he wrote in a letter to me:

> I noticed your book this past summer one day in a bookstore, and could not believe what perfect sense you made. I actually cut back on some of my exercise and added more fat to my diet. I applied your technology and the weight has been dropping off. I'm down to 205 now, and headed toward my ultimate goal of 174. On top of it all, I feel energized, whereas on every other diet, I always felt very drained. The Zone simply works.

Probably the best summary letter came from Len D.:

> I don't usually write fan mail, but after reading about your research results in the *New York Times*, I was intrigued enough to buy your book. To say that it was the best health investment I have ever made would be an understatement. As I read your book, I found myself wondering if you wrote it specifically for me. Your book was an epiphany for me, and it made such incredible sense. The body fat that I could not lose began melting away after about three days on the Zone Diet. The cravings disappeared, yet I found I could eat just three ounces of ice cream and not crave the rest of the carton. I haven't had real ice cream in years. This was incredible. At the risk of sounding overly dramatic, you have

been instrumental in returning control back to me, and it is such a powerful feeling that I felt compelled to write you to thank you personally. I may sound like a TV infomercial, but my energy has tripled, my clothes had to be taken in so they would fit, I'm sleeping better than I have in years and I am experiencing a profound change in the way I view food. Food is no longer a reward for me; I still love to eat, but food has become a necessary fuel to be mixed properly for maximum energy output. Your comparison of food to medicine is brilliant, yet so simple. Why didn't I make that connection? I wish you continued success in your crusade and please add my name to the list of individuals who have seen the light.

Obviously, I am very gratified when I receive such letters, testimonials, and profound thanks from people who feel I have changed their lives. But I tell these people that I did not change their lives; they did. I only provided them with the rules and tools to make the changes. They are the ones who really deserve all the credit. After hearing their stories, something may have struck a resonant note in your life.

I hope that some of these stories illustrate the potential of the Zone Diet to influence your health and your performance. It's not that the Zone Diet is revolutionary (after all, it is similar to what your grandmother recommended), it's just that it requires you to look at food hormonally, and take responsibility when you eat.

A small price to pay for SuperHealth.

16

TALES FROM THE OLYMPIC ZONE

Although the Zone Diet was developed to treat disease, the same hormonal control technology can dramatically improve athletic performance. The crucible for testing that statement occurs every four years at the Olympic Games.

One of the most important events in the development of the Zone Diet was its introduction to the Stanford University Swim Team coaches, Skip Kenney and Richard Quick, many years ago. Their willingness to commit their highly successful programs to a radically new dietary approach was a testimony to their belief that this technology could take their athletes to a higher level. In 1992, their faith was rewarded when Stanford swimmers won eight gold medals in Barcelona.

Four years later, in 1996, Richard and Skip were the U.S. Olympic Men's and Women's Head Coaches for swimming. Not surprising, considering that they have won eight out of the last ten NCAA Swimming Championships since integrating the Zone Diet into the men's and women's programs in 1992.

The 1996 Olympics in Atlanta proved no different from the 1992 Olympics. Another eight gold medals in swimming, just as in 1992.

In 1992 Jeff Rouse just missed Olympic gold in the 100-meter backstroke by a hundredth of a second. Vowing to return to the Olympics in 1996, for the next four years he remained the number one backstroker in the world. In Atlanta, he accomplished his goal and won the gold medal that had been just out of reach four years earlier. He also won another gold medal in the relays in Atlanta to go with a gold medal he won in relays in 1992, giving him a total of three gold medals and one silver medal for two Olympics.

Jenny Thompson completely dominated collegiate swimming during her four years at Stanford. In Atlanta, she won three gold medals to go with her two gold medals in Barcelona, making her the only U.S. woman ever to win that many Olympic gold medals in any sport. A Stanford teammate, Lisa Jacob, also won a gold medal in Atlanta.

Then there is Angel Martino, at age twenty-nine the oldest women ever to make the U.S. Olympic Swim Team. She qualified not just in one event, but in four. Angel's husband, Dr. Mike Martino, is an exercise physiologist who contacted me several years ago after he read about the Zone Diet and the Stanford swimmers, and said it made perfect sense. Since that time, Angel has trained without the benefit of an organized program, just her own will and the Zone Diet. Her results in Atlanta: two gold medals and two bronze medals.

But winning medals is not the only goal of the Olympics; it is the opportunity for the best of the world to compete. Just the opportunity to participate in the Olympics is the dream of any athlete. And that's why some of the other stories from Stanford are illuminating.

Take the case of Kurt Grote, who came to Stanford in 1992. At that time, he wasn't good enough to get a swimming scholarship. But in 1996 he made the U.S. Olympic Team, just about the highest achievement any swimmer can reach. Or the case of Ray Carey, who so severely damaged the nerve in his arm that doctors at Stanford said he would never swim again, let alone compete in the butterfly. Ray not only won the national championship last year, but, like Kurt, was a member of the 1996 Olympic Team.

These swimmers were not the only Zoners in the 1996 Olympics. Others included Alvin Harrison in track and field, who the previous year was so disappointed in his progress that he had stopped running. Once he went on the Zone Diet, his training was elevated to a new level and he renewed his commitment to making the Olympic team. At the Olympic Trials in June, he dropped a full second off his 400-meter times to make the team. The ending to his story was a gold medal in the 4 x 400–meter relay. And there is Sinjin Smith, a legend in beach volleyball, who was competing in Atlanta at the age of thirty-nine.

Were the diets of these elite athletes radically different from the diets of the people you heard from in the previous chapter? No. In fact, as I have already shown you, the diets are remarkably similar to those recommended for the typical American, except that these athletes require more protein and much more fat than the average person. In essence, within everyone's body lies the potential to at least look like an Olympic athlete, even if you cannot perform like one.

17

WHAT THE CRITICS SAY

I have come to realize that two things are very visceral in life: religion and nutrition. Both are based on belief systems instead of hard science. Science is never going to explain religion, but it can explain nutrition if you think hormonally. Frankly, there is no good diet or bad diet, only a hormonally correct one based on the foods a person will eat. What is my definition of a hormonally correct diet? One that keeps insulin in a tight zone, not too high or too low.

Many critics have called the Zone Diet a high-protein diet, which simply isn't true. It's a protein-adequate diet. Calling the Zone Diet a low-carbohydrate diet isn't correct, either. You are actually consuming more carbohydrates than protein on the Zone Diet. It's a carbohydrate-moderate diet. Calling the Zone Diet a high-fat diet also doesn't hold water. The actual total fat consumed on the Zone Diet is similar to that consumed in a typical vegetarian diet. A protein-adequate, carbohydrate-moderate, low-fat diet rich in fruits and vegetables; that's the definition of a Zone Diet. What I tried to put forward in *The Zone* is the scientific foundation for this kind of hormonal diet.

If you try to define a hormonally correct diet, then first you have to articulate the clinical criteria required to judge its success. I outlined these criteria in Chapter 12, but let me repeat them again. A hormonally correct diet is one that results in:

1. Loss of excess body fat (not just weight).
2. Increased energy and well-being.
3. A decrease in ratio of triglycerides to HDL cholesterol.
4. A decrease in fasting insulin.
5. A decrease in glycosylated hemoglobin.

Every one of these criteria has to be met before a diet can be called hormonally correct, since they all relate to the reduction of insulin levels. This is not a multiple-choice test. You have to achieve all of these simultaneously to have a hormonally correct diet.

And when it comes to determining if these criteria have been met, the blood tells all. Your blood doesn't have a political agenda. Whatever diet you are following, your blood levels will indicate whether you're maintaining a tight control on insulin and are therefore in the Zone. If you're controlling insulin, then by definition your diet is hormonally correct.

Since the publication of *The Zone,* other important studies have been published that further reinforce my concepts about the relationship of elevated insulin to cardiovascular disease. The first, which appeared in the *New England Journal of Medicine,* in 1996, showed that very slight elevations in fasting insulin levels made a significant difference in predicting who did or did not develop heart disease. A second appeared in *Coronary Artery Disease,* and concluded that the existence and severity of existing cardiovascular disease is strongly related to very slight increases in serum insulin. These studies support the basic tenet of *The Zone:* that elevated insulin is exceptionally dangerous to your health.

The tenet is also strongly supported by recent research from Harvard Medical School, first presented at the 1995 American Heart Association meeting, where a research report demonstrated that the ratio of triglycerides to HDL cholesterol is a powerful predictor of heart disease. This conclusion should not be surprising since elevated triglycerides and decreased HDL cholesterol levels both correlated to insulin resistance and hyperinsulinemia. In fact, this study indicated that patients with the higher triglyceride-to-HDL-cholesterol ratios were seventeen times more likely to have a heart attack than those with lower triglyceride-to-HDL-cholesterol ratios. A seventeen-times greater risk seems like a very good reason to keep your triglyceride-to-HDL-cholesterol ratio under tight control.

The relationship of obesity, insulin, and heart disease is now emerging more clearly. For example, a recent Harvard Medical School study published in 1995 demonstrated that if a woman gains more than fifteen to twenty pounds after the age of eighteen, she greatly increases her risk of heart disease. Now since this study was based on 115,000 nurses, the large sample size should carry some validity. That paper published in the *Journal of the American Medical Association* also stated that the new "1990 weight guidelines are falsely reassuring to the large proportion of women who are within current guidelines but have potentially avoidable increased risks of cardiovascular heart disease because of their weight."

Likewise, studies done at Stanford University have investigated the relationship between carbohydrate and fat intake and their effects on insulin by comparing different diets using overweight Type II diabetic patients (defined as being hyperinsulinemic). These patients do much better on a higher-fat (if it is monounsaturated fat) and lower-carbohydrate diet in controlled clinical trials, compared to the standard high-carbohydrate diets recommended to such patients. If a higher-fat, lower-carbohydrate diet is better for overweight, hyperinsulinemic Type II diabetic patients, then isn't it also better for overweight, hyperinsulinemic (but not yet Type II diabetic) Americans? I would say so.

Many of my critics often rely on epidemiological studies to support their case for consuming high-carbohydrate diets, insisting that any study (like those at the Stanford University Medical School) of less than one year in duration isn't meaningful, since it takes a long time for heart disease to develop. However, when considering epidemiological data about heart disease, I feel the only statistic that really counts is mortality. Viewing the data from the American Heart Association shown in Figures 17–1 and 17–2, you will see that the mortality rates from cardiovascular disease of different populations give rise to interesting paradoxes.

It is clear from each of these figures that the Japanese have a low rate of cardiovascular mortality. But then so do the French. And the French diet is very dissimilar to the Japanese diet. Is one diet superior to the other? I have eaten both, and enjoy both. And what about the Chinese, who eat a lot of rice, but not nearly as much animal protein (like fish) as the Japanese? If you study the urban Chinese (the ones who are not doing heavy physical labor that will reduce insulin levels), and compare them to Americans, you see very little difference in mortality rate. Therefore, broad statements that eating copious amounts of low-fat rice will prevent heart dis-

CVD Mortality Rates in Females Age 35-74

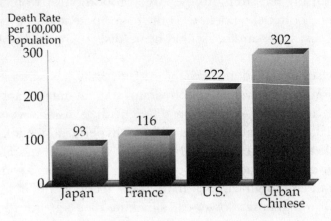

Figure 17-1. Cardiovascular Mortality Figures (Female)

CVD Mortality Rates in Males Age 35-74

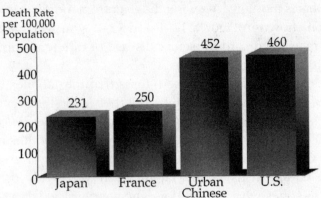

Figure 17-2. Cardiovascular Mortality Figures (Male)

ease may be true for urban Japanese, but not for urban Chinese.

What this really demonstrates is that epidemiological studies can be misleading. As Charles Hennekens of Harvard Medical School has said, "Epidemiology is a crude and inexact science. Eighty percent of the cases are almost hypotheses." The power of epidemiology is to identify a potential hypothesis from large-scale population studies to set up controlled clinical experiments to prove or disprove the hypothesis.

Support for the claims that high-carbohydrate diets are truly superior should come from long-term clinical studies in which the diet has been tightly controlled. To my knowledge, only one such study has been published, and that was in 1995. In this particular study, cardiovascular patients were maintained on a high-carbohydrate, vegetarian diet coupled with exercise and stress reduction for a five-year period.

Although the patients had better blood flow, their triglyceride/HDL cholesterol ratio (an indicator of insulin levels), which was high to begin with, had risen another 25 percent during the five-year period that the patients were on the high-carbohydrate, low-fat diet. And if you want to believe preliminary work from Harvard Medical School, the increase in the triglyceride-to-HDL-cholesterol ratio of these patients is not a healthy long-term situation. In fact, the lead author of that study, Dr. K. Lance Gould, a highly respected cardiologist, said in a 1996 letter in the *Journal of the American Medical Association*: "Frequently, triglyceride levels increase and HDL cholesterol levels decrease for individuals on vegetarian, high-carbohydrate diets. Since low HDL cholesterol, particularly with high triglycerides, incurs substantial risk of coronary events, I do not recommend a high-carbohydrate strict vegetarian diet."

All the research cited indicates the tide is slowly shifting toward the realization that the high-carbohydrate diet may not be the panacea for our ills that we were led to believe. But none of the research directly confirms that the Zone Diet is the direction in which we should be headed. Therefore one question about *The Zone* is justified, and that is the following: Has any independent study verified the results of the Zone Diet in hyperinsulinemic patients? Science is based on the ability of any investigator to repeat a study and get basically the same results. Until that replication has been done, a study done by the single investigator remains only suggestive. In *The Zone*, I presented data on hyperinsulinemic subjects that demonstrated significant clinical improvements following the Zone Diet for eight weeks, and even further clinical improvement at sixteen weeks. But has anyone reproduced that data? Isn't that the real question?

Fortunately, in February 1996, such a study was done and the results were reported in the *American Journal of Clinical Nutrition*. This study controlled the diet of forty-three overweight, hyperinsulinemic patients by confining them to a hospital ward for six weeks. The composition of the diet used in this study was essentially equivalent to the Zone Diet. During this study, the patients lowered their blood glucose, triglycerides, and insulin.

How did the results compare to the data I presented in *The Zone* that resulted from my study conducted with overweight, hyperinsulinemic, Type II diabetic patients? For comparison purposes, I have outlined various diets used in the study published by the *American Journal of Clinical Nutrition* and the study I conducted comparing the Zone Diet and a diet recommended by the American Diabetes Association (ADA). The data is presented in terms of the various protein-to-carbohydrate ratios. This ratio of protein to carbohydrate (i.e., your hormonal carburetor), which the Zone Diet is based upon, ideally should be 0.75. The results are shown in Table 16–1.

Table 16-1
Comparison of Protein-to-Carbohydrate (P/C) Ratios on Clinical Outcomes in Hyperinsulinemic Patients

P/C RATIO	GLUCOSE	INSULIN	TRIGLYCERIDES	TG/HDL
0.33 (ADA–8 weeks)*	−12%	+12%	+20%	+46%
0.64 (6 weeks)**	−7%	−8%	−18%	−12%
0.75 (Zone–8 weeks)*	−12%	−20%	−27%	−24%
0.75 (Zone–16 weeks)*	−15%	−30%	−35%	−30%

*From *The Zone* (1995), using Type II diabetic outpatients.
**From *American Journal of Clinical Nutrition* (1996), using metabolic ward patients.

As you can see from this table, changing the protein-to-carbo-hydrate ratio of a particular diet will alter insulin levels, and in turn lead to significant clinical improvement of blood glucose, triglyc-erides, and triglyceride-to-HDL-cholesterol ratio for the patients. And if you look at the clinical parameters, in particular the triglyc-eride-to-HDL-cholesterol ratio, the Zone Diet meets all the clinical criteria of a hormonally correct diet. And the longer the patients stayed on the Zone Diet, the better the clinical results.

If a growing body of research indicates something is wrong with our carbohydrate mania in treating overweight patients, why is it that the general population and vast majority of physicians still embrace the high-carbohydrate diet as the cure-all for our epidemic rise in obesity? One factor may be that the high-carbohydrate diet gives comfort if you're thinking calorically. After all, it's low in fat, and doesn't fat make you fat? And if fat is the enemy, then your bat-tle plan is to reduce all fat in the diet regardless of the type of fat.

On the other hand, if you are thinking hormonally, the high-car-bohydrate diet makes no sense whatsoever because it raises insulin levels in those who are genetically predisposed toward developing hyperinsulinemia or those who are already hyperinsulinemic. And it's increased insulin that not only makes you fat, but accelerates your progress toward heart disease. If insulin is the enemy, then your focus should be controlling the protein-to-carbohydrate ratio at every meal. There are two different potential enemies (fat versus insulin) and two different battle plans (a high-carbohydrate diet ver-sus a hormonally balanced diet). We have simply chosen the wrong enemy and the wrong battle plan for the past fifteen years.

The other factor that fuels this country's carbohydrate mania to keep Americans eating more and more carbohydrates is economics. One has to be realistic. There is a lot of money involved in pro-moting the high-carbohydrate diet. First, if you are a country pro-ducing millions of tons of wheat each year, what are you going to do with it? Animals won't eat it. The only thing wheat is good for is making bread, pasta, and bagels. And if you have a strong political lobby, you are going to do everything in your power to make sure the government encourages its citizens to buy as many wheat prod-ucts as possible. Maybe it's not so surprising that the base of the new U.S. food pyramid is composed primarily of wheat-based products. Also not surprisingly, consumption of pasta has increased by 115 percent in the past decade.

Second, if you're in the food manufacturing business, selling prepackaged carbohydrates makes excellent business sense. Protein is expensive, and fats go rancid. Given the opportunity to remove as much protein and fat as possible from packaged foods will improve shelf life and reduce costs. It makes good economic sense to do so. Furthermore, carbohydrates are dirt cheap, they last forever (remember pasta), they are politically correct, and they have the U.S. government seal of approval, plus billions of free advertising dollars to promote their consumption. It only makes sense to cater to this carbohydrate mania. And the sophistication of our food technology allows for virtually any product manufactured to consist primarily of carbohydrates.

Finally, the U.S. government, in an attempt to improve the health of the country, embraced a dietary concept (i.e., that eating more grain would decrease obesity) that was not well thought out in advance in terms of its hormonal consequences. It was a case of "shoot, ready, aim."

While there's no conspiracy to fatten Americans and make them less healthy, I do feel the convergence of these three trends (strong wheat lobby, profits in the food manufacturing sector, and government-driven "consensus") has been leading our country down a pathway toward a growing medical crisis.

And there is definite trouble lying ahead for the U.S. health care system. In early 1996, the American Heart Association announced that for the first time since 1980, deaths from cardiovascular disease are increasing. I'm afraid the hormonal chickens released during the last fifteen years of carbohydrate mania are coming home to roost.

Therefore, what is the best diet? It's one that you can stay on for the rest of your life and one that meets the clinical criteria I have outlined above. I believe that many of my critics will agree they are reasonable standards. Once we begin to treat nutrition as a science that can be judged by scientific standards, as opposed to some political or philosophical agenda, we as a country can get back to nutritional common sense.

What is desperately needed is a continuing dialog in this area as opposed to monolithic "consensus" based on belief systems.

Obviously, the belief system preached to Americans that carbohydrates (and especially pasta and bagels) are the essence of good nutrition simply isn't working well. Rather than preaching more of the same, doesn't it make sense to try other directions, like the one your grandmother used? I hope my critics agree.

One last thing about your grandmother. A recent study in the *New England Journal of Medicine* revealed which nationalities had the greatest longevity once they had reached the age of eighty, starting in 1960 and beyond. By 1995 they had obtained enough data to come to their conclusions. This data would likely have included your grandmother. And who had the greatest longevity? Was it the Japanese? No. Was it the French? No. Was it the Swedes? No. The answer was the Americans.

18

WHERE YOU GO FROM HERE

Every American should wake up to the new realities about access to unlimited, low-cost medical care in the twenty-first century. It's not going to exist, especially with the growing crisis in entitlement programs like Medicare. So you had better start planning now. In other words, your best health insurance policy is to achieve SuperHealth as quickly as possible.

As I stated in the beginning, SuperHealth is a state beyond health (if health is defined as the absence of disease). SuperHealth is about doing everything in your power to control hormonal levels and reduce the likelihood of developing chronic disease. That is what this book is all about, giving you the strategies to master the Zone.

You have to eat, so you might as well eat smart. Americans have the greatest potential to do this because we have the cheapest food in the world. Nonetheless, virtually no one in this country eats adequate levels of fruits and vegetables. Instead, we can't get enough fat-free, prepackaged goods. And in the process we are moving rapidly toward a medical abyss.

And if you don't care about yourself, think about your kids. Childhood obesity has increased by 50 percent over the last decade. At least give them a chance to get the most out of their lives. You control their food choices, because you buy and prepare their food. If you don't like what has happened to your own body composition and energy levels in the last fifteen years of carbohydrate gluttony, you at least experienced what it was like to have less body fat and greater energy in your youth. Give your kids the same chance.

In this book I have tried to give you as many helpful hints as possible to allow you to reorganize your dietary life. In reality, the adjustments are very easy: Just begin thinking hormonally. This is the big leap—moving away from caloric thinking to embrace hormonal thinking.

And once you understand hormonal thinking, it becomes clear that in the last fifteen years, we have lost all common sense as to what constitutes a good diet. Your grandmother knew it intuitively, but we have forgotten how to listen to her common sense.

What I'm hoping is that after reading this book, you will end up like one of the characters from the film *Network*, yelling at the top of your lungs, "I'm mad as hell, and I'm not going to take it anymore." Why should you be mad? Because many of you could have had a far better quality of life in the past fifteen years if only you had been given the correct information. And this information has been in the scientific peer-reviewed literature for decades. It was conveniently ignored because it didn't fit into a preconceived notion of a "correct diet." *You* have the ultimate control of your diet. Just use the commonsense rules given to you by your grandmother, and retake the driver's seat of your destiny.

Although *The Zone* was written to show a better way to treat chronic disease, I'm the first to realize that disease prevention is a pretty low priority for people in today's world. People often think only of "What's in it for me today?" Well, the Zone has that element, too. If you want to think better, perform better, and look better, then use the tools found in this book, and the concepts found in *The Zone*. All I ask is that you follow the program for two weeks. At the end of two weeks, if you're thinking better, performing better, and looking better, then stick with the program for another two weeks. At the end of four weeks, if you're still feeling good, try another two weeks. That's not much of a sacrifice.

What I hope to accomplish is to show you how nutrition can dramatically alter your life, if nutrition is based on the combination of science and common sense.

The twenty-first century will be the century in which people will finally learn to harness the most powerful drugs known: hormones. And in the era of hormonal control, the most powerful drug of all will be called food.

Your grandmother knew this. I hope that, after reading this book, you do too.

FURTHER RESOURCES

CONTINUING TECHNICAL SUPPORT

Free technical support is available from our Web site at http://www.Eicotech.com. Consider this Web site your Zone Community Center containing our on-line magazine with constantly updated medical research news, new Zone recipes, new Zone Diet tips, and answers to selected questions received by e-mail. Our Web site will also contain my recommendations about products and services that will help you get to and maintain yourself in the Zone. If you don't have access to a computer, then call our toll-free number at 800-550-6859 to obtain further technical information.

FOOD PRODUCTS

Wild Game

Wild game or range-fed beef and chicken are excellent sources of low-fat protein. Range-fed protein sources can be found in most high-quality supermarkets. Wild game can be obtained from specialty suppliers listed here:

Denver Buffalo Company
1120 Lincoln Street
Denver, CO 80203-970
Telephone: 800-289-2833

Game Exchange/Polarica
105 Quint Street
San Francisco, CA 94124
Telephone: 800-426-3872
or

73 Hudson Street
New York, NY 10013
Telephone: 800-426-3487

Soybean Products

Soybean products are excellent sources of plant-based protein. Imitation soybean meat products provide an excellent source of high-density vegetable protein. Information about more specialized sources of soybean products can be obtained from the following:

Soya Bluebook
P.O. Box 84
Bar Harbor, ME 04609

RECOMMENDED READING

The Zone
Barry Sears
ReganBooks, 1995

The basic reference text on which this book is based. *The Zone* goes into far greater detail about the biochemistry of hormonal control mechanisms of food and their effects on disease conditions.

Protein Power
Michael and Mary Dan Eades
Bantam, 1996

An excellent book on hyperinsulinemia written by close personal friends and longtime colleagues of mine. Since the underlying science in their book is the same as that found in *The Zone*, I strongly recommend it as a companion book to the Zone series. Although their initial dietary approach to reduce insulin starts with a higher protein-to-carbohydrate ratio than I recommend in *The Zone*, they gradually reintroduce carbohydrates to their patients so that their maintenance plan is the same as found in *The Zone*. We both agree that an individual has to adjust the protein-to-carbohydrate ratio to control insulin on a permanent basis.

Beyond Prozac
Michael Norden
ReganBooks, 1995

Written by an early pioneer in Prozac research, this book shows how simple interventions, including the Zone Diet, can increase serotonin levels (the pharmacological action of Prozac). An excellent resource for anyone interested in the effects and implications of serotonin-modulating drugs.

The Complete Book of Food Counts
Corinne T. Netzer
Dell, 1991

This book provides a listing of virtually every food product in terms of macronutrient composition. Convert each item into appropriate blocks, multiply the protein content of vegetable sources by 75 percent to get the amount of absorbable protein, and subtract the fiber content from the total carbohydrates to get the amount of insulin-promoting carbohydrate.

COMPUTER PROGRAMS

A number of inexpensive, good nutritional computer programs are on the market. While many more will be appearing, I recommend the following:

General Programs

Personal Chef 2.0 for Windows
    Parsons Technology
    One Parsons Drive
    Hiawatha, IA 52233-0100
    319-395-9626

Key Home Gourmet
    SoftKey International Corporation
    One Athenaeon Street
    Cambridge, MA 02142

Specific Zone Programs

These are specialty programs, especially designed for use with the Zone Diet.

The Zone Made Easy

Developed by Ted Wendler, this a useful program for determining body fat and block requirements, specifically based on *The Zone*. The program is available by calling 800-764-1019. Technical support for this program is available at 888-777-8839.

Zone Manager

A program developed by MetaMedix for automatically calculating Zone meals based on your protein requirements, using your favorite foods. The program contains over 5,000 foods to plan your meals, and you can add your own foods or recipes. This program is available by calling 800-455-4105. Technical support for this program is available at 800-684-3015.

FOOD BLOCKS

The concept of macronutrient food blocks gives a straightforward method to construct Zone meals. Listed below are the portion sizes of blocks of proteins, carbohydrates, and fats equal to one block. Note that the protein volumes are for uncooked portions. Each carbohydrate block represents the amount of insulin-promoting carbohydrate in that portion size. Although favorable carbohydrates are usually low-glycemic carbohydrates, there are exceptions (like ice cream and potato chips) that are also high in fat (see Glycemic Index in Appendix E).

I have rounded off the blocks to convenient sizes for easy memory. This list is by no means meant to be exhaustive. If you have a favorite food that is not listed, simply refer to Corinne Netzer's *Complete Book of Food Counts* (Dell, 1991) to expand the list. This list has been updated since the publication of *The Zone,* and as a result some block sizes have been altered from my original version.

When constructing a Zone meal, always remember the primary rule: Keep the protein and carbohydrate blocks in a 1:1 ratio.

PROTEIN BLOCKS (APPROXIMATELY 7 GRAMS PROTEIN PER BLOCK)

Meat and Poultry

Best Choices (low in saturated fat)

Beef (range-fed or game)	1 ounce
Chicken breast, skinless	1 ounce
Chicken breast, deli-style	1½ ounces
Turkey breast, skinless	1 ounce
Turkey breast, deli-style	1 ounce

Fair Choices (moderate in saturated fat)

Beef, lean cuts	1 ounce
Canadian bacon, lean	1 ounce
Chicken, dark meat, skinless	1 ounce
Corned beef, lean	1 ounce
Duck	1½ ounces
Ham, lean	1 ounce
Ham, deli-style	1½ ounces
Hamburger (less than 10 percent fat)	1½ ounces
Lamb, lean	1 ounce
Pork, lean	1 ounce
Pork chop	1 ounce
Turkey bacon	3 strips
Turkey, dark meat, skinless	1 ounce
Veal	1 ounce

Poor Choices (high in either saturated fat or arachidonic acid or both)

Bacon, pork	3 strips
Beef, fatty cuts*	1 ounce
Beef, ground (10 to 15 percent fat)	1½ ounces
Beef, ground (more than 15 percent fat)*	1½ ounces
Hot dog (pork or beef)	1 link
Hot dog (turkey or chicken)	1 link
Kielbasa	2 ounces
Liver, beef*	1 ounce
Liver, chicken*	1 ounce
Pepperoni	1 ounce
Salami	1 ounce

*Contains arachidonic acid.

Fish and Seafood

Bass	1 ounce
Bluefish	1 ounce
Calamari	2½ ounces

Catfish	1½ ounces
Clams	1½ ounces
Cod	1½ ounces
Crabmeat	1½ ounces
Haddock	1½ ounces
Halibut	1½ ounces
Lobster	1 ounce
Mackerel**	1½ ounces
Salmon**	1½ ounces
Sardine**	1 ounce
Scallops	1½ ounces
Shrimp	1½ ounces
Snapper	1½ ounces
Swordfish	1½ ounces
Trout	1 ounce
Tuna (steak)	1 ounce
Tuna, canned in water	1 ounce

**Rich in EPA.

Eggs

Best Choices

Egg whites	2
Egg substitute	¼ cup

Fair Choices

Cheese, non-fat	1 ounce
Whole egg*	1

*Contains arachidonic acid.

Protein-Rich Dairy

Best Choices

Cottage cheese, low-fat	¼ cup

Fair Choices

Cheese, reduced-fat	1 ounce
Mozzarella cheese, skim	1 ounce
Ricotta cheese, skim	2½ ounces

Poor Choice

Hard cheeses	1 ounce

Protein-Rich Vegetarian

Tofu, firm and extra-firm	3 ounces
Protein powder	⅓ ounce
Soy burgers	½ patty
Soy hot dog	1 link
Soy sausages	2 links
Soy sausage	1 patty

Mixed Protein/Carbohydrate (contains one block of protein and one block of carbohydrate)

Milk, low-fat (1 percent)	1 cup
Soy flour	⅓ cup
Tempeh	1½ ounces
Tofu, soft and regular	3 ounces
Yogurt, plain	½ cup

CARBOHYDRATE BLOCKS (APPROXIMATELY 9 GRAMS OF INSULIN-PROMOTING CARBOHYDRATE PER BLOCK)

Favorable Carbohydrates

Cooked Vegetables

Artichoke	1 medium
Asparagus	1 cup (12 spears)
Beans, green or wax	1 cup
Beans, black	¼ cup
Bok choy	3 cups

Broccoli	1¼ cups
Brussels sprouts	1½ cups
Cabbage, shredded	1⅓ cups
Cauliflower	2 cups
Chickpeas	¼ cup
Collard greens, chopped	2 cups
Eggplant	1½ cups
Kale	1¼ cups
Kidney beans	¼ cup
Leeks	1 cup
Lentils	¼ cup
Mushrooms (boiled)	1 cup
Okra, sliced	1 cup
Onions, chopped (boiled)	¾ cup
Sauerkraut	1 cup
Spinach, chopped	1¼ cups
Swiss chard, chopped	1½ cups
Turnip, mashed	1 cup
Turnip greens, chopped	1¾ cups
Yellow squash (summer), sliced	1¼ cups
Zucchini, sliced	1½ cups

Raw Vegetables

Alfalfa sprouts	11 cups
Bamboo shoots, cuts	1¼ cups
Broccoli	1½ cups
Cabbage, shredded	3 cups
Cauliflower, pieces	2 cups
Celery, sliced	2½ cups
Cucumber	1
Cucumber, sliced	4 cups
Endive, chopped	7½ cups
Escarole, chopped	7½ cups
Green or red peppers	3
Green pepper, chopped	2¼ cups
Humus	¼ cup
Lettuce, iceberg (six-inch diameter)	1 head

Lettuce, romaine, chopped	4 cups
Mushrooms, chopped	3 cups
Onion, chopped	1 cup
Radishes, sliced	2½ cups
Salsa	½ cup
Snow peas	1 cup
Spinach, chopped	6 cups

Spinach salad (3 cups raw spinach,
   ¼ raw onion,
   ¼ raw mushrooms,
   and ¼ raw tomato)
	1

Tomato	2
Tomato, chopped	1¼ cups

Tossed salad (2 cups shredded lettuce,
   ¼ raw green bell pepper,
   ¼ raw cucumber,
   and ¼ raw tomato)
	1

Water chestnuts	⅓ cup

Fruits (fresh, frozen, or canned light)

Apple	½
Applesauce	⅓ cup
Apricots	3
Blackberries	¾ cup
Blueberries	½ cup
Boysenberries	¾ cup
Cantaloupe	¼ melon
Cantaloupe, cubed	¾ cup
Cherries	¾ cup
Fruit cocktail	½ cup
Grapefruit	½
Grapes	½ cup
Honeydew melon, cubed	½ cup
Kiwi fruit	1
Lemon	1
Lime	1
Nectarine, medium	½

Orange	½
Orange, mandarin, canned	⅓ cup
Peach	1
Peaches, canned	½ cup
Pear	½
Pineapple, cubed	½ cup
Plum	1
Raspberries	1 cup
Strawberries	1 cup
Tangerine	1
Watermelon, cubed	¾ cup

Grains

Barley (dry)	½ tablespoon
Oatmeal (slow-cooking)***	⅓ cup (cooked)
Oatmeal (slow-cooking)***	½ ounce dry

***Contains GLA.

Unfavorable Carbohydrates (use in moderation)

Cooked Vegetables

Acorn squash	½ cup
Baked beans	⅛ cup
Beets, sliced	½ cup
Butternut squash	½ cup
Carrot	1
Carrot, shredded	1 cup
Carrot, sliced	½ cup
Corn	¼ cup
French fries	5
Lima beans	¼ cup
Parsnip	⅓
Peas	⅓ cup
Pinto beans	¼ cup
Potato, baked	⅓ cup
Potato, boiled	⅓ cup
Potato, mashed	⅕ cup

Refried beans	¼ cup
Sweet potato, baked	⅓
Sweet potato, mashed	⅕ cup

Fruits

Banana	⅓
Cranberries, chopped	¾ cup
Cranberry sauce	3 teaspoons
Dates	2 pieces
Fig	1 piece
Guava	½ cup
Kumquat	3
Mango, sliced	⅓ cup
Papaya, cubed	¾ cup
Prunes (dried)	2
Raisins	1 tablespoon

Fruit Juices

Apple	⅓ cup
Apple cider	⅓ cup
Cranberry	¼ cup
Fruit punch	¼ cup
Grape	¼ cup
Grapefruit	⅓ cup
Lemon	⅓ cup
Lemonade	⅓ cup
Orange	⅓ cup
Pineapple	¼ cup
Tomato	1 cup
V–8	¾ cup

Grains, Cereals, and Breads

Bagel (small)	¼
Biscuit	½
Bread crumbs	½ ounce

Bread, whole grain	½ slice
Bread, white	½ slice
Breadstick, soft	½
Breadstick, hard	1
Buckwheat, dry	½ ounce
Bulgur wheat, dry	½ ounce
Cereal, dry	½ ounce
Cornbread	one-inch square
Cornstarch	1 teaspoon
Couscous, dry	1 ounce
Cracker, saltine	4
Cracker, Triscuit	3
Croissant, plain	½
Crouton	½ ounce
Doughnut, plain	¾
English muffin	¼
Granola	½ ounce
Grits, cooked	⅓ cup
Melba toast	½ ounce
Millet	½ ounce
Muffin, blueberry	½
Noodles, egg (cooked)	¼ cup
Pancake (four-inch)	½
Pasta, cooked	¼ cup
Pita bread	¼ pocket
Pita bread, mini	½ pocket
Popcorn, popped	2 cups
Rice, brown (cooked)	⅕ cup
Rice, white (cooked)	⅕ cup
Rice cake	1
Roll, bulkie	¼
Roll, dinner	½ small
Roll, hamburger	½
Taco shell	1 small
Tortilla, corn (six-inch)	1
Tortilla, flour (eight-inch)	½
Waffle	½

Alcohol

Beer	6 ounces
Distilled spirits	1 ounce
Wine	4 ounces

Others

Barbecue sauce	2 tablespoons
Candy bar	¼
Cake	⅓ slice
Cocktail sauce	2 tablespoons
Cookie (small)	1
Crackers (saltine)	4
Crackers (graham)	1½ pieces
Honey	½ tablespoons
Ice cream, regular	¼ cup
Ice cream, premium	⅙ cup
Jam or jelly	2 tablespoons
Ketchup	2 tablespoons
Molasses, light	1½ teaspoons
Plum sauce	1½ tablespoons
Potato chips	½ ounce
Pretzels	½ ounce
Relish, pickle	4 teaspoons
Sugar, brown	2 teaspoons
Sugar, granulated	2 teaspoons
Sugar, confectionery	1 tablespoon
Syrup, maple	2 teaspoons
Syrup, pancake	2 teaspoons
Teriyaki sauce	1 tablespoon
Tortilla chips	½ ounce

FAT BLOCKS (APPROXIMATELY 1.5 GRAMS OF FAT PER BLOCK)

Best Choices (rich in monounsaturated fat)

Almond butter	⅓ teaspoon
Almonds (slivered)	1½ teaspoon

Almonds (whole)	3
Avocado	1 tablespoon
Canola oil	⅓ teaspoon
Guacamole	1 tablespoon
Macadamia Nut	1
Olive oil	⅓ teaspoon
Olive oil and vinegar dressing (⅓ teaspoon olive oil and ⅔ teaspoons vinegar)	1 teaspoon
Olives	3
Peanut butter, natural	½ teaspoon
Peanut oil	⅓ teaspoon
Peanuts	6
Tahini	½ teaspoon

Fair Choices (low in saturated fat)

Mayonnaise, regular	⅓ teaspoon
Mayonnaise, light	1 teaspoon
Sesame oil	½ teaspoon
Soybean oil	⅓ teaspoon
Walnuts, shelled and chopped	1 teaspoon

Poor Choices (rich in saturated fat)

Bacon bits (imitation)	1½ teaspoons
Butter	⅓ teaspoon
Cream (half-and-half)	1 tablespoon
Cream cheese	1 teaspoon
Cream cheese, light	2 teaspoons
Lard	⅓ teaspoon
Sour cream	½ tablespoon
Sour cream, light	1 tablespoon
Vegetable shortening	⅓ teaspoon

APPENDIX C

CALCULATION OF LEAN BODY MASS

A rapid way to determine your lean body mass is simply to use a tape measure and scale. You should make all measurements on bare skin (not through clothing), and make sure that the tape fits snugly but does not compress the skin and underlying tissue. Take all measurements three times and calculate the average. All measurements should be in inches. The tables used to calculate the percentage of body fat were used with the permission of Dr. Michael Eades from his book *Thin So Fast*.

Calculating Body-Fat Percentages for Females

There are five steps you must take to calculate your percentage of body fat:

1. While keeping the tape level, measure your hips at their widest point, and your waist at the umbilicus (i.e., belly button). It is critical that you measure at the belly button and not at the narrowest point of your waist. Take each of these measurements three times and compute the average.
2. Measure your height in inches without shoes.
3. Record your height, waist, and hip measurements on the accompanying worksheet.
4. Find each of these measurements in the appropriate column in the accompanying tables and record the constants on the worksheet.
5. Add Constants A and B, then subtract Constant C for this sum and round to the nearest whole number. That figure is your percentage of body fat.

Worksheet for Women to Calculate Their Percentage of Body Fat

Average hip measurement _____ (used for Constant A)

Average abdomen measurement _____ (used for Constant B)

Height _____ (used for Constant C)

Using Table 1, look up each of the average measurements and your height in the appropriate column.

$$\text{Constant A} = \underline{\hspace{2cm}}$$

$$\text{Constant B} = \underline{\hspace{2cm}}$$

$$\text{Constant C} = \underline{\hspace{2cm}}$$

To determine your approximate percentage of body fat, then add Constant A and B. From that total, subtract Constant C. The result is your percentage of body fat.

Calculating Body-Fat Percentages for Men

There are four steps you must take to determine your body-fat percentage:

1. While keeping the tape level, measure the circumference of your waist at the umbilicus (i.e., belly button). Measure three times and compute the average.
2. Measure your wrist at the space between your dominant hand and your wrist bone, at the location where your wrist bends.
3. Record these measurements on the worksheet for males.
4. Subtract your wrist measurement from your waist measurement and find the resulting value listed in the table. On the left-hand side of this table, find your weight. Proceed to right from your weight and down from your waist-minus-wrist measurement. Where these two points intersect, read your body fat percentage.

Worksheet for Men to Calculate Their Percentage of Body Fat

Average waist measurement _____ (inches)

Average wrist measurement _____ (inches)

Subtract the wrist measurement from the waist measurement. Use Table 2 to find your weight. Then find your "waist minus wrist" number. Where the two columns intersect is your approximate percentage of body fat.

Calculating Lean Body Mass for Both Females and Males

Now that you know your body-fat percentage, the next step is to use this figure to calculate the weight in pounds of the fat portion of your total body weight. This is done by multiplying your weight by your percentage of body fat. (Remember to use a decimal point—15 percent is 0.15 for example.)

(Weight) × (% of body fat) = total body-fat weight

Once you know the weight of your total body fat, you subtract that total fat weight from your total weight, which results in your lean body mass. Lean body mass is the total weight of all nonfat body tissue.

_____ Your total weight

− _____ Your total of body fat

= _____ Your lean body mass

Lean body mass = total weight − total body-fat weight

TABLE 1

CONVERSION CONSTANTS FOR PREDICTION OF PERCENTAGE OF BODY FAT IN FEMALES

Hips		Abdomen		Height	
Inches	Constant A	Inches	Constant B	Inches	Constant C
30	33.48	20	14.22	55	33.52
30.5	33.83	20.5	14.40	55.5	33.67
31	34.87	21.0	14.93	56	34.13
31.5	35.22	21.5	15.11	56.5	34.28
32	36.27	22	15.64	57	34.74
32.5	36.62	22.5	15.82	57.5	34.89
33	37.67	23	16.35	58	35.35
33.5	38.02	23.5	16.53	58.5	35.50
34	39.06	24	17.06	59	35.96
34.5	39.41	24.5	17.24	59.5	36.11
35	40.46	25	17.78	60	36.57
35.5	40.81	25.5	17.96	60.5	36.72
36	41.86	26	18.49	61	37.18
36.5	42.21	26.5	18.67	61.5	37.33
37	43.25	27	19.20	62	37.79
37.5	43.60	27.5	19.38	62.5	37.94
38	44.65	28	19.91	63	38.40
38.5	45.32	28.5	20.27	63.5	38.70
39	46.05	29	20.62	64	39.01
39.5	46.40	29.5	20.80	64.5	39.16
40	47.44	30	21.33	65	39.62
40.5	47.79	30.5	21.51	65.5	39.77
41	48.84	31	22.04	66	40.23
41.5	49.19	31.5	22.22	66.5	40.38
42	50.24	32	22.75	67	40.84
42.5	50.59	32.5	22.93	67.5	40.99
43	51.64	33	23.46	68	41.45
43.5	51.99	33.5	23.64	68.5	41.60
44	53.03	34	24.18	69	42.06
44.5	53.41	34.5	24.36	69.5	42.21
45	54.53	35	24.89	70	42.67

Hips		Abdomen		Height	
Inches	Constant A	Inches	Constant B	Inches	Constant C
45.5	54.86	35.5	25.07	70.5	42.82
46	55.83	36	25.60	71	43.28
46.5	56.18	36.5	25.78	71.5	43.43
47	57.22	37	26.31	72	43.89
47.5	57.57	37.5	26.49	72.5	44.04
48	58.62	38	27.02	73	44.50
48.5	58.97	38.5	27.20	73.5	44.65
49	60.02	39	27.73	74	45.11
49.5	60.37	39.5	27.91	74.5	45.26
50	61.42	40	28.44	75	45.72
50.5	61.77	40.5	28.62	75.5	45.87
51	62.81	41	29.15	76	46.32
51.5	63.16	41.5	29.33		
52	64.21	42	29.87		
52.5	64.56	42.5	30.05		
53	65.61	43	30.58		
53.5	65.96	43.5	30.76		
54	67.00	44	31.29		
54.5	67.35	44.5	31.47		
55	68.40	45	32.00		
55.5	68.75	45.5	32.18		
56	69.80	46	32.71		
56.5	70.15	46.5	32.89		
57	71.19	47	33.42		
57.5	71.54	47.5	33.60		
58	72.59	48	34.13		
58.5	72.94	48.5	34.31		
59	73.99	49	34.84		
59.5	74.34	49.5	35.02		
60	75.39	50	35.56		

TABLE 2
MALE PERCENTAGE BODY FAT CALCULATIONS

Waist-Wrist (in inches)	22	22.5	23	23.5	24
Weight (in lbs.)					
120	4	6	8	10	12
125	4	6	7	9	11
130	3	5	7	9	11
135	3	5	7	8	10
140	3	5	6	8	10
145		4	6	7	9
150		4	6	7	9
155		4	5	6	8
160		4	5	6	8
165		3	5	6	8
170		3	4	6	7
175			4	6	7
180			4	5	7
185			4	5	6
190			4	5	6
195			3	5	6
200			3	4	6
205				4	5
210				4	5
215				4	5
220				4	5
225				3	4
230				3	4
235				3	4
240					4
245					4
250					4
255					3
260					3
265					
270					
275					
280					
285					
290					
295					
300					

24.5	25	25.5	26	26.5	27	27.5
14	16	18	20	21	23	25
13	15	17	19	20	22	24
12	14	16	18	20	21	23
12	13	15	17	19	20	22
11	13	15	16	18	19	21
11	12	14	15	17	19	20
10	12	13	15	16	18	19
10	11	13	14	16	17	19
9	11	12	14	15	17	18
9	10	12	13	15	16	17
9	10	11	13	14	15	17
8	10	11	12	12	15	16
8	9	10	12	13	14	16
8	9	10	11	13	14	15
7	8	10	11	12	13	15
7	8	9	11	12	13	14
7	8	9	10	11	12	14
6	8	9	10	11	12	13
6	7	8	9	11	12	13
6	7	8	9	10	11	12
6	7	8	9	10	11	12
6	7	8	9	10	11	12
5	6	7	8	9	10	11
5	6	7	8	9	10	11
5	6	7	8	9	10	11
5	6	7	8	9	9	10
5	6	6	7	8	9	10
4	5	6	7	8	9	10
4	5	6	7	8	9	10
4	5	6	7	8	8	9
4	5	6	7	7	8	9
4	5	5	6	7	8	9
4	4	5	6	7	8	9
4	4	5	6	7	8	8
3	4	5	6	7	7	8
3	4	5	6	6	7	8
3	4	5	5	6	7	8

Waist-Wrist (in inches)	28	28.5	29	29.5	30	30.5	31
Weight (in lbs.)							
120	27	29	31	33	35	37	39
125	26	28	30	32	33	35	37
130	25	27	28	30	32	34	36
135	24	26	27	29	31	32	34
140	23	24	26	28	29	31	33
145	22	23	25	27	28	30	31
150	21	23	24	26	27	29	30
155	20	22	23	25	26	28	29
160	19	21	22	24	25	27	28
165	19	20	22	23	24	26	27
170	18	19	21	22	24	25	26
175	17	19	20	21	23	24	25
180	17	18	19	21	22	23	25
185	16	18	19	20	21	23	24
190	16	17	18	19	21	22	23
195	15	16	18	19	20	21	22
200	15	16	17	18	19	21	22
205	14	15	17	18	19	20	21
210	14	15	16	17	18	19	21
215	13	15	16	17	18	19	20
220	13	14	15	16	17	18	19
225	13	14	15	16	17	18	19
230	12	13	14	15	16	17	18
235	12	13	14	15	16	17	18
240	12	13	14	15	16	17	17
245	11	12	13	14	15	16	17
250	11	12	13	14	15	16	17
255	11	12	13	14	14	15	16
260	10	11	12	13	14	15	16
265	10	11	12	13	14	15	15
270	10	11	12	13	13	14	15
275	10	11	11	12	13	14	15
280	9	10	11	12	13	14	14
285	9	10	11	12	12	13	14
290	9	10	11	11	12	13	14
295	9	10	10	11	12	13	14
300	9	9	10	11	12	12	13

31.5	32	32.5	33	33.5	34	34.5
41	43	45	47	49	50	52
39	41	43	45	46	48	50
37	39	41	43	44	46	48
36	38	39	41	43	44	46
34	36	38	39	41	43	44
33	35	36	38	39	41	43
32	33	35	36	38	40	41
31	32	34	35	37	38	40
30	31	33	34	35	37	38
29	30	31	33	34	36	37
28	29	30	32	33	34	36
27	28	29	31	32	33	35
26	27	28	30	31	32	34
25	26	28	29	30	31	33
24	26	27	28	29	30	32
24	25	26	27	28	30	31
23	24	25	26	28	29	30
22	23	25	26	27	28	29
22	23	24	25	26	27	28
21	22	23	24	25	26	28
20	22	23	24	25	26	27
20	21	22	23	24	25	26
19	20	21	22	23	24	25
19	20	21	22	23	24	25
18	19	20	21	22	23	24
18	19	20	21	22	23	24
18	18	19	20	21	22	23
17	18	19	20	21	22	23
17	18	19	19	20	21	22
16	17	18	19	20	21	22
16	17	18	19	19	20	21
16	16	17	18	19	20	21
15	16	17	18	19	19	20
15	16	17	17	18	19	20
15	15	16	17	18	19	19
14	15	16	17	17	18	19
14	15	16	16	17	18	19

Waist-Wrist (in inches)	35	35.5	36	36.5	37
Weight (in lbs.)					
120	54				
125	52	54			
130	50	52	53	55	
135	48	50	51	53	55
140	46	48	49	51	53
145	44	46	47	49	51
150	43	44	46	47	49
155	41	43	44	46	47
160	40	41	43	44	46
165	38	40	41	43	44
170	37	39	40	41	43
175	36	37	39	40	41
180	35	36	37	39	40
185	34	35	36	38	39
190	33	34	35	37	38
195	32	33	34	35	37
200	31	32	33	35	36
205	30	31	32	34	35
210	29	30	32	33	34
215	29	30	31	32	33
220	28	29	30	31	32
225	27	28	29	30	31
230	26	27	28	30	31
235	26	27	28	29	30
240	25	26	27	28	29
245	25	26	27	27	28
250	24	25	26	27	28
255	24	24	25	26	27
260	23	24	25	26	27
265	22	23	24	25	26
270	22	23	24	25	25
275	22	22	23	24	25
280	21	22	23	24	24
285	21	21	22	23	24
290	20	21	22	23	23
295	20	21	21	22	23
300	19	20	21	22	22

37.5	38	38.5	39	39.5	40	40.5
54						
52	54	55				
50	52	53	55			
49	50	52	53	55		
47	48	50	51	53	54	
45	47	48	50	51	52	54
44	45	47	48	49	51	52
43	44	45	47	48	49	51
41	43	44	45	47	48	49
40	41	43	44	45	46	48
39	40	41	43	44	45	46
38	39	40	41	43	44	45
37	38	39	40	41	43	44
36	37	38	39	40	41	43
35	36	37	38	39	40	42
34	35	36	37	38	39	40
33	34	35	36	37	38	39
32	33	34	35	36	37	38
32	33	34	35	36	37	38
31	32	33	34	35	36	37
30	31	32	33	34	35	36
29	30	31	32	33	34	35
29	30	31	31	32	33	34
28	29	30	31	32	33	34
27	28	29	30	31	32	33
27	28	29	29	30	31	32
26	27	28	29	30	31	31
26	27	27	28	29	30	31
25	26	27	28	29	29	30
25	26	26	27	28	29	30
24	25	26	27	27	28	29
24	25	25	26	27	28	28
23	24	25	26	26	27	28

Waist-Wrist (in inches)	41	41.5	42	42.5	43	43.5
Weight (in lbs.)						
120						
125						
130						
135						
140						
145						
150						
155						
160						
165	55					
170	54	55				
175	52	53	55			
180	50	52	53	54		
185	49	50	51	53	54	55
190	48	49	50	51	52	54
195	46	47	49	50	51	52
200	45	46	47	48	50	51
205	44	45	46	47	48	49
210	43	44	45	46	47	48
215	42	43	44	45	46	47
220	41	42	43	44	45	46
225	40	41	42	43	44	45
230	39	40	41	42	44	44
235	38	39	40	41	42	43
240	37	38	39	40	41	42
245	36	37	38	39	40	41
250	35	36	37	38	39	40
255	34	35	36	37	38	39
260	34	35	35	36	37	38
265	33	34	35	36	36	37
270	32	33	34	35	36	37
275	32	32	33	34	35	36
280	31	32	33	33	34	35
285	30	31	32	33	34	34
290	30	31	31	32	33	34
295	29	30	31	32	32	33
300	29	29	30	31	32	33

44	44.5	45	45.5	46	46.5	47
55						
53	55					
52	53	54	55			
51	52	53	54	55		
49	50	51	53	54	55	
48	49	50	51	52	53	54
47	48	49	50	51	52	53
46	47	48	49	50	51	52
45	46	47	48	49	50	51
44	45	46	47	48	49	50
43	44	45	46	46	47	48
42	43	44	44	45	46	47
41	42	43	44	44	45	46
40	41	42	43	44	44	45
39	40	41	42	43	43	44
38	39	40	41	42	43	43
37	38	39	40	41	42	43
37	38	38	39	40	41	42
36	37	38	38	39	40	41
35	36	37	38	39	39	40
35	35	36	37	38	39	39
34	35	36	36	37	38	39
33	34	35	36	36	37	38

Waist-Wrist (in inches)	47.5	48	48.5	49	49.5	50
Weight (in lbs.)						
120						
125						
130						
135						
140						
145						
150						
155						
160						
165						
170						
175						
180						
185						
190						
195						
200						
205						
210						
215	55					
220	54	55				
225	53	54	55			
230	52	53	54	55		
235	51	51	52	53	54	55
240	49	50	51	52	53	54
245	48	49	50	51	52	53
250	47	48	49	50	51	52
255	46	47	48	49	50	51
260	45	46	47	48	49	50
265	44	45	46	47	48	49
270	43	44	45	46	47	48
275	43	43	44	45	46	47
280	42	43	43	44	45	46
285	41	42	43	43	44	45
290	40	41	42	43	43	44
295	39	40	41	42	43	43
300	39	39	40	41	42	43

Day in the Zone Meal Construction Template

Breakfast

	Protein	Carbohydrate	Added Fat
Protein Course			
Main Carb. Course			
Total			

Lunch

	Protein	Carbohydrate	Added Fat
Salad			
Protein Course			
Main Carb. Course			
Dessert			
Alcohol			
Total			

Dinner

	Protein	Carbohydrate	Added Fat
Salad			
Protein Course			
Main Carb. Course			
Dessert			
Alcohol			
Total			

APPENDIX E

GLYCEMIC INDEX

Terms such as "simple" and "complex" carbohydrates are meaningless when it comes to reaching the Zone. What really matters to the body is the amount and the rate at which a carbohydrate enters into the bloodstream (which in turn determines the extent of insulin secretion). The body is extremely efficient in absorbing carbohydrates so that all the carbohydrate that you consume will eventually enter the bloodstream. This is why controlling the overall amount of carbohydrate in a meal is critical. However, the rate at which the carbohydrate component of a particular food is converted to glucose and enters the blood can be variable. This rate of carbohydrate entry into the bloodstream is known as the glycemic index. Foods that contain no carbohydrate will not have a glycemic index.

To determine a glycemic index of a food, usually 50 grams of insulin-promoting carbohydrate (subtracting the fiber content from the total carbohydrate content) is given to a test subject. Blood sugar levels are carefully and periodically monitored over the next three hours, and the response curve is plotted. The response to the reference food is tested at least three times and the results are averaged.

From these time points, the area under the response curve for the test food is expressed as a percent of the mean value for the reference food (e.g., white bread) for the same subject. The percentages from several subjects are then averaged together to obtain the glycemic index for any particular food. The higher the glycemic index for a food, the faster it will raise blood sugar levels, and therefore increase insulin secretion.

The actual glycemic index of a food is a number relative to the standard of white bread, which is given a glycemic index of 100. Although the glycemic index of a food is fairly standard, the insulin response of an individual to a defined amount of carbohydrate entering the bloodstream can be highly variable.

The glycemic index is also affected by the way a food is prepared. Greater processing of the food results in a breakdown of the cell walls, allowing the carbohydrates in a food to be broken down faster into simple sugars for absorption. This is why refried beans have a much higher glycemic index than kidney beans. In addition, fat will always decrease the glycemic index of a given carbohydrate because the fat content will decrease the rate of carbohydrate absorption into the blood. This is why potato chips have a lower glycemic index than potatoes, even though they have been highly processed.

The glycemic index is a valuable tool to help determine which carbohydrates will most likely get you to the Zone. Regardless of the glycemic index of a food, never consume more carbohydrate blocks from that food in a meal than protein blocks. It is the ratio of the protein to carbohydrate that is the primary determining factor to get you to the Zone. The glycemic index should be viewed as a broad guide to help you choose more favorable carbohydrates in constructing your Zone meals. Within a particular grouping, each food is ranked in order of its measured glycemic index.

GLYCEMIC INDEX OF FOODS BASED ON THE RATE OF ENTRY INTO THE BLOODSTREAM

Extremely high (greater than 100)

Grain-based foods
　　Puffed rice
　　Cornflakes
　　Millet
　　Rice, instant
　　Potato, instant
　　Bread, French

Vegetables
Parsnips, cooked
Potato, russet, baked
Potato, instant
Carrots, cooked
Broad beans (Fava beans)

Simple sugars
Maltose
Glucose
Honey

Glycemic Standard=100 percent
Bread, white

High (80–100)

Grain-based foods
Bread, wheat, whole meal
Grapenuts
Tortilla, corn
Shredded wheat
Muesli
Bread, rye, crispbread
Bread, rye, whole meal
Rice, brown
Porridge oats
Corn, sweet
Rice, white

Vegetables
Potato, mashed
Potato, new, boiled

Simple sugars
Sucrose

Fruits
Apricots
Raisins
Banana

Papaya
Mango

Snacks
Corn chips
Mars Bar
Crackers
Cookies
Pastry
Ice cream, low-fat

Moderately high (60–80)

Grain-based foods
Buckwheat
All Bran
Bread, rye, pumpernickel
Bulgur
Macaroni, white
Spaghetti, white
Spaghetti, brown

Vegetables
Yam
Potato, sweet
Green peas, marrowfat
Green peas, frozen
Baked beans (canned)
Kidney beans (canned)

Fruits
Fruit cocktail
Grapefruit juice
Orange juice
Pineapple juice
Pears, canned
Grapes

Snacks
Cookies, oatmeal
Potato chips
Sponge cake

Moderate (40–60)

Vegetables
Haricot (white) beans
Tomato soup
Brown beans
Lima beans
Green peas, dried
Chickpeas (garbanzo)
Butter beans
Black-eyed peas
Kidney beans
Black beans

Fruits
Orange
Apple juice
Pears
Apple

Dairy
Yogurt
Ice cream, high-fat
Whole milk
2 percent milk
Skim milk

Low (less than 40)

Grain-based food
Barley

Vegetables
Red lentils
Soybeans, canned
Soybeans, dried

Fruits
    Peaches
    Plums

Simple sugars
    Fructose

Snacks
    Peanuts

APPENDIX F

REFERENCES

American Heart Association. "Heart and Stroke Facts: 1996 Statistical Supplement."

_____. "Heart Disease and Strokes Deaths Rising." January 24, 1996, press release.

Anderson, G.H. "Metabolic Regulation of Food Intake." In *Modern Nutrition in Health and Disease*, edited by M.E. Shils and V.R. Young, 557-569. Philadelphia: Lea and Febiger, 1988.

Bao, W., S.R. Srinivasan, and G.S. Berenson. "Persistent Elevation of Plasma Insulin Levels Is Associated with Increased Cardiovascular Risk in Children and Young Adults." *Circulation* 93 (1996): 54–59.

Bidoli, E., S. Franceschi, R. Talamini, S. Barra, and C. La Vecchia. "Food Consumption and Cancer of the Colon and Rectum in North-Eastern Italy." *International Journal of Cancer* 50 (1992): 223–229.

Blum, M., M. Auerbuch, V. Wolman, and A. Aviram. "Protein Intake and Kidney Function in Humans: Its Effect on Normal Aging." *Archives Internal Medicine* 149 (1989): 211–212.

Blundell, J.E., and V.J. Burley. "Evaluation of the Satiating Power of Dietary Fat in Man." In *Progress in Obesity Research*, edited by Y. Onumura, 453–457. New York: John Libbey, 1990.

Brothwell, D., and A.T. Sandison, eds. *Diseases in Antiquity: A Survey of the Disease.* Springfield, Ill.: C.C. Thomas, 1967.

Brunning, P.F., J.M.G. Bonfrer, P.A.H. van Noord, A.A.M. Hart, M. de Jong-Bakker, and W.J. Nooijen. "Insulin Resistance and Breast Cancer Risk." *International Journal of Cancer* 52 (1992): 511–516.

Chen, Y.I., A.M. Coulston, M. Zhou, C.B. Hollenbeck, and G.M. Reaven. "Why Do Low-Fat High-Carbohydrate Diets Accentuate Postprandial Lipemia in Patients with NIDDM?" *Diabetes Care* 18 (1995): 10–16.

Cockburn, A., and E. Cockburn, eds. *Mummies, Disease, and Ancient Cultures.* Cambridge, England: Cambridge University Press, 1980.

Corti, M-C., J.M. Guraink, M.E. Saliva, T. Harris, T.S. Field, R.B. Wallace, L.F. Berkman, T.E. Seeman, R.J. Glynn, C.H. Hennekens, and R.J. Havlik. "HDL Cholesterol Predicts Coronary Heart Disease Mortality in

Older Persons." *Journal of the American Medical Association* 274 (1995): 539–544.

Crawford, M., and D. Marsh. *The Driving Force: Food, Evolution and the Future.* New York: Harper and Row, 1989.

Despres, J.P., B. Lamarche, P. Mauriege, B. Cantin, G.R. Dagenais, S. Moorjani, and P.J. Lupen. "Hyperinsulinemia as an Independent Risk Factor for Ischemic Heart Disease." *New England Journal of Medicine* 334 (1996): 952–957.

Drexel, H., F.W. Amann, J. Beran, K. Rentsch, R. Candinas, J. Muntwyler, A. Leuthy, T. Gasser, and F. Follath. "Plasma Triglycerides and Three Lipoprotein Cholesterol Fractions Are Independent Predictors of the Extent of Coronary Atherosclerosis." *Circulation* 90 (1994): 2230–2235.

Eades, M., and M.D. Eades. *Protein Power.* New York: Bantam, 1996.

Eaton, S.B. "Humans, Lipids, and Evolution." *Lipids* 27 (1992): 814–820.

Eaton, S.B., and M.J. Konner. "Paleolithic Nutrition." *New England Journal of Medicine* 312 (1985): 283–289.

Eaton, S.B., M. Konner, and M. Shostalle. "Stone Agers in the Fast Lane: Chronic Degenerative Diseases in Evolutionary Implications." *American Journal of Medicine* 84 (1988): 739–749.

Eaton, S.B., M. Shostalle, and M. Konner. *The Paleolithic Prescription.* New York: Harper and Row, 1988.

Flatt, J-P. "Use and Storage of Carbohydrate and Fat." *American Journal of Clinical Nutrition* 61 (1995): 952S–959S.

Fontbonne, A., G. Tchobroutsky, E. Eshwege, J.L. Richard, J.R. Claude, and G.E. Rosselin. "Coronary Heart Disease Mortality Risk; Plasma Insulin Level Is a More Sensitive Marker Than Hypertension or Abnormal Glucose Tolerance in Overweight Males." *International Journal of Obesity* 12 (1988): 557–565.

Franceschi, S., A. Favero, A. Decarli, E. Negri, C. La Vecchia, M. Ferranroni, A. Russo, S. Salvini, D. Amadori, E. Conti, M. Montella, and A. Giacosa. "Intake of Macronutrients and Risk of Breast Cancer." *Lancet* 347 (1996): 1351–1356.

Garg, A., J.P. Bantle, R.R. Henry, A.M. Coulston, and G.M. Reaven. "Effects of Varying Carbohydrate Content of Diet in Patients with Non-Insulin Dependent Diabetes Mellitus." *Journal of the American Medical Association* 271 (1994): 1421–1428.

Gaziano, M., and C. Hennekens. "Triglycerides, HDL, and Risk of Myocardial Infarction in a Case-Control Study." Abstract presented at the annual meeting of the American Heart Association, Anaheim, CA, November 1995.

Golay, A., A.F. Allaz, Y. Morel, N. de Tonnac, S. Tankova, and G. Reaven. "Similar Weight Loss with Low- or High-Carbohydrate Diets." *American Journal of Clinical Nutrition* 63 (1996): 174–178.

Gould, K.L. "Very Low-Fat Diets for Coronary Heart Disease: Perhaps, but Which One?" *Journal of the American Medical Association* (1996) 275: 1402–1403.

Gould, K.L., D. Ornish, L. Scherwitz, S. Brown, R.P. Edens, M.J. Hess, N. Mullani, L. Bolomey, F. Dobbs, W.T. Armstrong, T. Merritt, T. Ports, S. Sparier, and J. Billings. "Changes In Myocardial Perfusion Abnormalities by Positron Emission Tomography After Long-Term, Intense Risk Factor Modification." *Journal of the American Medical Association* 274 (1995): 894–901.

Hollenbeck, C., and G.M. Reaven. "Variations in Insulin-Stimulated Glucose Uptake in Healthy Individuals with Normal Glucose Tolerance." *Journal of Clinical Endocrinology and Metabolism* 64 (1987): 1169–1173.

Holt, S., J. Brand, C. Soveny, and J. Hansky. "Relationship of Satiety to Postprandial Glycemic, Insulin, and Cholecystokinin Responses." *Appetite* 18 (1992): 129–141.

Hunt, J.R., S.K. Gallagher, L.K. Johnson, and G.I. Lykken. "High versus Low-Meat Diets: Effects on Zinc Absorption, Iron Status, and Calcium, Copper, Iron, Magnesium, Manganese, Nitrogen, Phosphorous, and Zinc Balance in Postmenopausal Women." *American Journal of Clinical Nutrition* 62 (1995): 621–632.

Jiang, W., M. Babyak, D.S. Krantz, R.A. Waugh, E. Coleman, M.M. Hanson, D.J. Frid, S. McNulty, J.J. Morris, C.M. O'Connor, and J.A. Blumenthal. "Mental Stress-Induced Myocardial Ischemia and Cardiac Events." *Journal of the American Medical Association* (1996) 275: 1651–1656.

Job, F.P., J. Wolfertz, R. Meyer, A. Hubinger, F.A. Gries, and H. Kuhn. "Hyperinsulinism in Patients with Coronary Artery Disease." *Coronary Artery Disease* 5 (1994): 487–492.

Karhapaa, P., M. Malkki, and M. Laakso. "Isolated Low HDL Cholesterol: An Insulin-Resistant State." *Diabetes* 43 (1994): 411–417.

Kekwick, A., and G.L.S. Pawan. "Calorie Intake in Relation to Body-Weight Changes in the Obese." *Lancet* 2 (1956): 155–161.

———. "Metabolic Study in Human Obesity with Isocaloric Diets High in Fat, Protein or Carbohydrate." *Metabolism* 6 (1957): 447–460.

Klarhr, S., A.S. Levey, G.J. Beck, A.W. Caggiula, L. Hunsicker, J.W. Kusek, and G. Striker. "The Effects of Dietary Protein Restriction and Blood-Pressure Control on the Progression of Chronic Renal Disease." *New England Journal of Medicine* 330: (1994) 877–884.

La Vecchia, C., E. Negri, A. Decarli, B. D'Avanzo, and S. Franceschi. "A Case-Control Study of Diet and Gastric Cancer in Northern Italy." *International Journal of Cancer* 40 (1992): 484–489.

Laws, A., A.C. King, W.L. Haskell, and G.M. Reaven. "Relation of Fasting Plasma Insulin Concentration to High-Density Lipoprotein Cholesterol and Triglyceride Concentrations in Men." *Arteriosclerosis and Thrombosis* 11 (1991): 1636–1642.

Leek, F.F. "Dental Health and Disease in Ancient Egypt with Special Reference to the Manchester Mummies." In *Science in Egyptology*, edited by R.A. Davis, 35–42. Manchester, England: Manchester University Press, 1986.

Mallick, N.P. "Dietary Protein and Progression of Chronic Renal Disease: Large Randomized Controlled Trial Suggests No Benefit from Restriction." *British Medical Journal* 309 (1994): 1101–1102.

Manton, K.G., and J.W. Vaupel. "Survival After Age of 80 in the United States, Sweden, France, England, and Japan." *New England Journal of Medicine* 333 (1995): 1232–1235.

Miller, M., A. Seidler, P.O. Kwiterovich, and T.A. Pearson. "Long-Term Predictors of Subsequent Cardiovascular Events with Coronary Artery Disease and 'Desirable' Levels of Plasma Total Cholesterol." *Circulation* 86 (1992): 1165–1170.

Modan, M., H. Halkin, J. Or, A. Karasik, Y. Drory, Z. Fuchs, A. Lusky, and A. Chetrit. "Hyperinsulinemia, Gender and Risk of Atherosclerotic Cardiovascular Disease." *Circulation* 84 (1991): 1165–1175.

Norman, A.W., and G. Litwack. *Hormones*. New York: Academic Press, 1987.

Oates, J.A., G.A. FitzGerald, R.A. Branch, E.K. Jackson, H.R. Knapp, and L.J. Roberts. "Clinical Implications of Prostaglandin and Thromboxane A_2 Formation. Part 1." *New England Journal of Medicine* 319 (1988): 689–698.

———. "Clinical Implications of Prostaglandin and Thromboxane A_2 Formation. Part 2." *New England Journal of Medicine* 319 (1988): 761–767.

Paffenbarger, R.S., and W.E. Hale. "Physical Activity as an Index of Heart Attack Risk in College Alumni." *American Journal of Epidemiology* 108 (1978): 161–175.

Paffenbarger, R.S., R.T. Hyde, A.L. Wing, and C. Hsieh. "Physical Activity, All-Cause Mortality, and Longevity of College Alumni." *New England Journal of Medicine* 314 (1986): 613–615.

Parillo, M., A.A. Rivellese, A.V. Ciardul, B. Capaldo, A. Giacco, S. Genovese, and G. Riccardi. "A High Monounsaturated-Fat/Low-

Carbohydrate Diet Improves Peripheral Insulin Sensitivity in Non-Insulin-Dependent Diabetic Patients." *Metabolism* 41 (1992): 1373–1378.

Patch, J.R., G. Miesenbock, T. Hopferwieser, V. Muhlberger, E. Knapp, J.K. Dunn, A.M. Gotto, and W. Patsch. "Relation of Triglyceride Metabolism and Coronary Artery Disease." *Arteriosclerosis and Thrombosis* 12 (1992): 1336–1345.

Phinney, S.D., P.G. Davis, S.B. Johnson, and R.T. Holman. "Obesity and Weight Loss Alter Polyunsaturated Metabolism in Humans." *American Journal of Clinical Nutrition* 52 (1991): 831–838.

Phinney, S.D., R.S. Odin, S.B. Johnson, and R.T. Holman. "Reduced Aracidonate in Serum Phospholipids and Cholesteryl Esters Associated with Vegetarian Diets in Humans." *American Journal of Clinical Nutrition* 51 (1991): 385–392.

Puech, P.F., and F.F. Leek. "Dental Microwear As an Indication of Plant Food in Early Man." In *Science in Egyptology*, edited by R.A. Davis, 239–242. Manchester, England: Manchester University Press, 1986.

Pyorala, K., E. Savolainen, S. Kaukula, and J. Haapakoski. "Plasma Insulin As Coronary Heart Disease Risk Factor." *Acta Med Scandinavia* 701 (1985): 38–52.

Reaven, G.M. "Role of Insulin Resistance in Human Disease." *Diabetes* 37 (1988): 1595–1607.

_____. "The Role of Insulin Resistance and Hyperinsulinemia in Coronary Heart Disease." *Metabolism* 41 (1992): 16–19.

Remer, T., and F. Manz. "Dietary Protein As a Modulator of the Renal Net Acid Excretion Capacity: Evidence That an Increased Protein Intake Improves the Capability of the Kidney to Excrete Ammonium." *Nutritional Biochemistry* 6 (1995): 431–437.

Renauld, S., and M. De Lorgeril. "Wine, Alcohol, Platelets and the French Paradox for Coronary Heart Disease." *Lancet* 339 (1992): 1523–1528.

Schapira, D.V., N.B. Kumar, G.H. Lyman, and C.E. Cox. "Abdominal Obesity and Breast Cancer Risk." *Ann Int Medicine* 112 (1990): 182–186.

Schwartz, M.W., D.P. Figlewicz, D.G. Baskin, S.C. Woods, and D. Porte. "Insulin in the Brain: A Hormonal Regulator of Energy Balance." *Endocrine Review* 13 (1992): 387–414.

Sears, B. *The Zone*. New York: HarperCollins, 1995.

Serra-Majem, L., L. Ribas, R. Tresserras, and L. Salleras. "How Could Changes in Diet Explain Changes in Coronary Heart Disease Mortality in Spain? The Spanish Paradox." *American Journal of Clinical Nutrition* 61 (1995): 1351S–1359S.

Silver, M.J., W. Hoch, J.J. Kocsis, C.M. Ingerman, and J.B. Smith.

"Arachidonic Acid Causes Sudden Death in Rabbits." *Science* 183 (1974): 1085–1087.

Smith, N.J.D. "Dental Pathology in an Ancient Egyptian Population." In *Science in Egyptology*, edited by R.A. Davis, 43-48. Manchester, England: Manchester University Press, 1986.

Spencer, H., L. Kramer, M. DeBartolo, C. Morris, and D. Osis. "Further Studies of the Effect of a High Protein Diet As Meat on Calcium Metabolism." *American Journal of Clinical Nutrition* 37 (1983): 924–929.

Spencer, H., L. Kramer, and D. Osis. "Do Protein and Phosphorus Cause Calcium Loss?" *Journal of Nutrition* 118 (1988): 657–660.

United States Department of Agriculture. *Research News.* January 16, 1996.

Wellborn, T.A., and K. Wearne. "Coronary Heart Disease Incidence and Cardiovascular Mortality in Busselton with Reference to Glucose and Insulin Concentrations." *Diabetes Care* 2 (1979): 154–160.

Willett, W.C., J.E. Manson, M.J. Stampfer, G.A. Colditz, B. Rosner, F.E. Speizer, and C.H. Hennekens. "Weight, Weight Change, and Coronary Heart Disease in Women." *Journal of the American Medical Association* 273 (1995): 461–465.

Wolever, T.M.S., D.J.A. Jenkins, A.L. Jenkins, and R.G. Josse. "The Glycemic Index: Methodology and Clinical Implications." *American Journal of Clinical Nutrition* 54 (1991): 846–854.

Wu, D., S.N. Meydani, M. Meydani, M.G. Hayek, P. Huth, and R.J. Nicolosi. "Immunologic Effects of Marine- and Plant-Derived N–3 Poly-unsaturated Fatty Acids in Nonhuman Primates." *American Journal of Clinical Nutrition* 63 (1996): 273–280.

Young, V.R., and P.L. Pellett. "Plant Proteins in Relation to Human Protein and Amino Acid Nutrition." *American Journal of Clinical Nutrition* 59 (1994): 1203–1212S.

GENERAL INDEX

ACE (angiotensin-converting enzyme) inhibitors, 283
adrenaline, 282
alcohol, 18–19, 38
almonds, 24, 37, 269, 297
alpha linolenic acid (ALA), 293
American Diabetes Association, 312
American Heart Association, 308, 314
    cardiovascular mortality figures, 310
American Journal of Clinical Nutrition, 312
appetite. *See* CCK; hunger
arachidonic acid, 23, 292, 295
athletes
    elite, 9, 31, 306
    fat requirements, 30–31
    protein requirements for, 7–8, 31, 58
    week of meals, female, 83–96
    week of meals, male, 96–108
    and Zone diet, 288, 304–6
avocado/guacamole as source of dietary fat, 24, 37, 297

bagels, 3, 17, 284, 315. *See also* carbohydrates, unfavorable
beef, hormones and antibiotics in, 288
block method (of portion control), 6, 290
    carbohydrates, 15–16, 26, 33
    fat, 24, 26, 33–34, 292–93
    and nutritional labels, 264
    protein, 5–6, 26, 33
    ratio, 25–26, 292–93, 294
blood
    diagnostic testing, 276–77
    pressure and hyperinsulinemia, 276
    pressure and Zone diet, 300
    sugar levels, 29, 274
    types and insulin response, 44–45
breakfast. *See also* meals, on Zone Diet
    cereal, 18, 264–66
    timing, 48, 52

business trips, eating during, 272–73

caffeine, 283
calcium intake, 287
calories, 28
    amount stored, average, 29, 285
    classic study of low-, diet, 28, 285
    and high carbohydrate diet, 313
    low intake, 284–85
    per meal, 37
    and Zone Diet, 29, 313
    Zone rule on, 270
cancer
    prevention, 50
    surviving, and Zone diet, 299
carbohydrate
    blocks, 15–16, 26, 33
    consumption, 10, 15
    cooking and absorption, 290
    cravings, 4, 54, 56, 286, 302
    as a drug, 273
    and eating out, 271–73
    and fat intake, 21
    favorable/unfavorable, 16, 35, 48, 51, 55, 284, 289, 290
    high carbohydrate diets, 3, 291, 311–12, 313
    and insulin, 12, 15, 17, 21, 275
    quick list, 14–15
    ratio to protein, 25–26, 264, 294
    too little, 46
    too much, 45–46, 275
    total intake, 285–86
    types of, 11, 26
    unfavorable, maximum intake, 48, 289
    Zone rules on, 14, 19, 20
Carey, Ray, 305
chewing food, 57
chicken, hormones and antibiotics in, 288

RECIPE INDEX